RETROSPECTIVE WELLNESS SERIES

BOOK I

YOUR GUIDE TO A LONG & HEALTHY LIFE

SRIPREMRAJ SINNAIAH

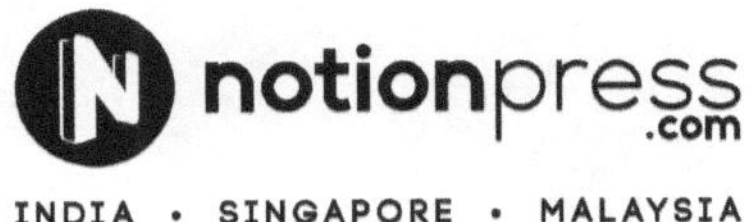

Notion Press

Old No. 38, New No. 6
McNichols Road, Chetpet
Chennai - 600 031

First Published by Notion Press 2020

ISBN 978-1-64850-862-2

Dedication

Dedicated to all those bravehearts fighting battles for better health.

Contents

Preface

Believe in the Afterlife?

Do you believe in the afterlife? Depending on the individual's belief there will be 'Yes' or 'No' but one thing is for certain: this is the only life where you will live with the same consciousness, which means you have only one life to live. If it's the only chance, I would say you give your best shot at it. Giving the best shot at life means doing what you feel like doing, relishing every occasion, converting events into sweet memories, making friends, having more adventures, and most importantly when you look back at your life at the inevitable moment of your life's end you shouldn't feel the tiniest form of regret. To make it possible you should be at your prime health condition throughout your life and the more time you have, the merrier it is. So longevity signifies extending your time in this world as long as you enjoy prime health during your stay.

During my childhood, I grew up with more fun and celebration rather than fear. I was surrounded by parents, friends, their families, and everyone who filled my life with happiness than any other emotions. As a boy, all my fears were limited only to school assignments, losing a sports game or similar trivial issues. Those were the days where I would welcome the flu or cough or some form of illness that can get me a day off from school. But things have changed; Look at the condition now: there is one constant fear lurking in everyone's mind and even though most people don't admit it, it is the fear of sickness. Nowadays, people are paranoid over bouts of simple flu infections. Whether it is them or their kids or their family who gets infected, everyone is in a state of fear. For all the advancement in the field of medicine, surprisingly, people's fear of sickness has only increased. In my view, this is a very sad situation that needs to be addressed immediately.

I decided to write this book to give hope to people, instil confidence, better their lives, remind them of a few basic principles that we have forgotten over the recent years, and finally empower them to celebrate life at its best. After all, we have just one life and it will be a pity to waste it over a fear of illness. In this book, I have thrown some light on methods one can follow to improve one's chance of a beautiful life.

I do acknowledge the fact that in the past two decades, we have seen so many outbreaks of diseases and the terrible part is not the sickness but the panic that creates among people. All around the world, people take extra measures to keep their house safe from any attack from external elements, natural or otherwise. If we can do so much for a house, why can't we fight for our lives against various forms of illness? To my surprise, in recent times people's mindset has changed so much that they lose confidence in themselves at the first sign of an attack and surrender themselves to the oppressor or they immediately seek external aid. The trouble in seeking external aid is that half of the masses don't know when will the help arrive or even worse, it could be another form of attack. In this book, I have given insight into methods with which they can stand their ground against any form of attack and believe in their capabilities. An attack could mean any form of illness or disease. At the end of this book, I believe people will be more sophisticated with the right set of tools and also have more confidence in themselves to handle any kind of sickness—both physical and mental. If you are one of those who would like to put up a fight when your health is under attack, then this book will prove very helpful.

If you have reached this far, that means you have made up your mind to spend a precious part of your time reading my book and I assure you won't regret it. Let's start from the beginning. Whatever concepts I have included in this book hold good for humans irrespective of their gender, race, ethnicity or any other diversifying factor.

Longevity

Longevity, literally, means living longer, but it also means much more than that. There is no point in extending your lifespan by lying in a bed, unable to perform your basic duties and always needing external assistance. Nor is it better to have a life full of regrets without enjoying even small happiness. On a broader view, longevity means a person living his life to the fullest or rather I would say celebrating his time on this planet until his last breath. I know most of us think: "It is usually easier said than done." In recent times with the advancement of technologies, most of us believe things blindly rather than analyze data. The difference between the two is that the fact is the data has been proved right and accepted. Longevity has become one of the most sought out treasure. The wealthy invest their resources while the poor invest their hope on it. And I am sure this quest for conquering longevity will continue as long as we exist. This is my sincere effort to explain longevity in the simplest form possible.

Several factors influence this entity. Some of the prominent factors include gender, location, race and lifestyle. This is one of the key phenomena, which have taken up a large amount of time and resources in the forms of various researches. From the time humans came to be in existence, there has been a lot of effort put in to understand and manipulate this particular process. That's because nobody wants to die. With the evolution of human intelligence, they have come to understand the fact that there is simply not enough time for everyone to do all the things they intend to do during their lifetime. This realization led to the concept called longevity. In recent times, the evolution of things around us is tremendously fast and we humans are forced to sacrifice things that matter. Take Steve Jobs, one of the most successful people. He fought against many battles in life to reach the top but ultimately lost the fight against cancer at a relatively young age. Who knows what else he could have achieved if he had been alive for a few more years and how people's lives could have become even better with his newer inventions. That's just one famous instance I have mentioned here; there are, of course, millions of such inspiring examples are all around us if you start looking deep provided you have the time. But the notion of this book is not to give you a case study. All that matters is the realization that irrespective of your wealth and power, health is the single most important thing a person should be looking at any point of life.

'Health is Wealth' is an age-old saying, which holds good almost to all classes of people from different walks of life and at all times.

None in the world can counter this simple but profound statement. Being healthy doesn't end with having good health for a particular period and after that one falls sick and succumbs to the suffering that takes away your peace and your loved ones' as well. In the contemporary world, 'Health is everything' should be the new motto.

There are several types of research revolving around the health field and hundreds of proved facts in the form of research papers and experiments. Nevertheless, there are always some individuals who triumph over others when it comes to living longer than the average expectancy of a person. How do they do that? It is the focus of numerous researches done in the past, present and future also. Maybe it is because of this reason most of the books and articles on health provide a specific set of solutions for specific health conditions: like considering a particular herb or follow a specific diet or a particular exercise routine for a particular health condition. Nothing wrong about it, honestly, I would also be looking at a set of articles and books, which are relevant to my health condition. It is human nature or rather human intelligence to look out for solutions that have triggered our evolution among all the other species on this planet. The feat we have achieved so far is beyond comparison with any other living species on this planet. But all I can tell you is that there is an overload of information available in the recent items that have made us blind to the underlying basic principles.

Basic principles are relatively very simple but extremely effective when applied in its original form. Like any other science subject, human health also has a set of basic underlying principles, which needs to be understood to apply later on in one's life. It is like having a manual to a machine that has been there all this while on our table but we never realized the value of it. When I started discussing the idea of writing a book on longevity, a good friend of mine countered with a really valuable question. "There are already more than enough sources of information about any kind of health condition; what is the significance of this book?"

It got me thinking and then I figured out a satisfying answer—There is simply too much information for any common man to digest and people get lost in this ocean of information. However, despite this overwhelming information, people are still searching for an answer. This is similar to the scenario of what happens if someone drops you in the middle of the ocean without life support, even if you possess the capabilities of the Olympic swimmer, Michael Phelps, you won't survive for long and you will eventually drown. You need directions to get yourself out of this condition.

Likewise, in this book, I have taken efforts to establish a concept-wise approach to achieve longevity based on examples and knowledge acquired from various medical studies backed up by researches and my experiences. I will be setting forth some basic principles that I believe governs human health. These principles would act as a piece of guiding equipment, giving directions towards long-lasting health. The moment people understand how this works, they will be able to manipulate their path towards longevity. It is like identifying your route to your destination with GPS.

Let us look at an interesting fact about age classifications. There are a few definitions for old age classifications available but one classification inspired me to include it here. It is as below:

- 65–74—Young-Old

- 75–84—Middle-Old

- 85—Old-Old

As per this, a person can be considered old only when he crosses 85 years of age, but in our contemporary society reaching 80 years with good health is a humongous task and seldom does anyone dreams of life after 85. Even if someone is strong enough to cross

85, his happiness depends primarily on his physical health condition leaving aside his relationships, financial status and other factors. Ironically, we are living in an age where we have made unimaginable advancements in medical sciences, but the average lifespan of a human in the present times is only 79. We will be forced to imagine death as a phenomenon, which is single-handedly taking this whole world with its inventions (i.e. diseases) and relentless efforts despite so many advancements we make in medical sciences every day. This is saddening.

Acknowledging the fact that we are advancing at a rapid rate in both human health and recovery, our mortality rate is also increasing rapidly. We should remind ourselves of another fact – when we look into our past most of the people cruised through their old age without the need for any of the modern medicines or sophisticated machines, which are run by artificial intelligence. They didn't have any of our medicines, devices or scope. In fact, they had almost nothing when compared to our multi-speciality hospital facilities. What does that signify? If we devote a part of our efforts spent on inventing new medicines looking at our past generations and researching their way of life, we could avoid several medical complications, and in certain cases death also. All it takes is just a bit of effort in terms of discovering the way of life in our previous generations and belief in what our forefathers followed. If you start digging deep inside our previous generations and their lifestyles, the facts are very real; humans can live a longer, happier and healthier life. All these are just data and we need a leap of faith to understand that. All that we need is available right around us and we don't get to see them. Maybe at the end of this book, you will be empowered to see those things.

Mathematics Behind Longevity

Mathematics is an interesting adventure for those who love it and obstinate trouble for those who don't. I am one of the latter; nevertheless, I did find out that the most complex part of mathematics is understanding the simple point that every mathematical problem can be solved by a combination of addition and subtraction. For that matter, the other two basic mathematic principles being multiplication and division are just repeated addition and repeated subtraction, respectively. Any mathematics professor will agree on this. You have to trust me when I say that there is no problem in the world that you can't solve with these two processes, the only difference is the number of repetitions that we need for a particular issue. A primary school kid uses simple additions and subtractions, whereas a graduate uses the same additions and subtractions in the form of complex formulas, rules and concepts. The underlying magic lies within the two processes only. But the point to remember would be that each problem will have its solution with a specific number of steps, you can't solve all the problems with the same set of steps.

When a person can analyze a set of similar problems and establishes a specific set of these steps, it becomes a formula. Some formulas can be used to solve a problem and some to make the process more efficient. So the next time when the problem falls into one of the already defined categories, we get to use the pre-defined formulas. This process has continued from the time mathematics has been in use. Since this spans into a few centuries, most of us tend to overlook the underlying principle that addition and subtraction are still the fundamental processes. Now, the relationship of this concept to this book is quite simple and a few might have already understood the reason.

Similar to the mathematical problems, we face a lot of problems with our health and the pre-defined formulas become medicines and the ones who prescribe it to us become the doctor. A few formulas like wellness concepts are used for the betterment of health. As per the ancient Indian medicinal science, there are over 4000+ known diseases and not all the diseases had a cure at that time (even now we don't have cures for a few fatal ones). So in those days, the wise ones with futuristic vision understood this and have explained the basic underlying principles for a healthy life in a unique way. Quite interestingly, if you analyze different cultures among people, they have certain specific habits imbibed in their day-to-day life without really understanding the importance of that. I have tried to explain these simple but effective lifestyle choices in this book that have been the secret of our forefathers' healthy and peaceful life.

My Intriguing Vacation

Let me tell you an incident, which has lots of relevance to the concepts in this book. When I was a kid, my family used to visit my uncle who lives in the hills. The house was situated on the slopes of a hill surrounded by tea plantations. It was lush and surrounded by amazing scenic beauty! The mere thought of the place is enough to bring me out of any form of stress. The interesting part is that there was no clearly defined path to reach the house. Every time we had to wander around trying to find our path among the tea shrubs. It takes climbing down and up a few hills, slopes to reach the road with transportation facilities. Once in a while, we end up returning in the latter part of the day and the place used to be completely covered in darkness because there were no streetlights from the actual road to my uncle's house. Who would want to light up the way to an individual's house? Even if wanted to, there were very few houses spaced at roughly half a kilometre in the middle of the hills. If you ever stayed in any hill resort, you will know what I mean. During the night, my uncle used to lead the way, and he could do so without needing any light, whereas I used to struggle even with a torch in my hand. Frequently, I used to get lost in the darkness. Mostly, my uncle will come to my rescue and will guide me through the path.

Initially, I thought the problem was with the torch and so every time I visited his house I used to take a bigger torch, so much so that I finally ended up taking a lamp, one of the recent inventions during my childhood, to solve this puzzle. But irrespective of the type of light source used, I never really made any real progress in finding my route to my uncle's house on my own. Having run out of options, I once asked my uncle how he is able to find the way even in the pitch dark without any light. He asked me to wait till nightfall and then took me out to a spot around a kilometre away from the house into the middle of nowhere. Suddenly, he left my hand and started walking back. Taken by surprise, I called out to him saying I didn't bring any torch along. He didn't care to reply to me and kept walking. I desperately tried to follow him in vain. In moments he disappeared into the darkness and I was all alone in the middle of a hill with darkness covering me like a blanket. I was really scared and my mind was racing through available options: screaming was the easiest, but my uncle has always warned me about screaming in the middle of the night, which will attract unnecessary attention from the wild animals. So I desperately waited for my uncle to come back and find me. After around two minutes, a miracle happened and I realized what my uncle was trying to convey.

My eyes slowly got adjusted to the darkness giving me the ability to find my way in the middle of darkness guided by the light from the moon and stars. That was the last time I ever got lost in the middle of hills in the night. Even though the stars and moon were there from the beginning, the torch or torches I used during my attempts made me blind to this fact and instead it gave me the ability to see only a few yards. With every bigger torch, I was able to cover a bigger but limited area, while all I had to do was switch off the light to see the whole distance.

My takeaway from this incident is that the older generations were able to find their way towards longevity without the need for any advanced technologies while we try to retrace the same path with all the recent technologies just like me trying to find the path with a better torch. All that we have to do is take a leap back into the past with faith and look out for the path towards longevity.

Giving Back Longevity

Recently I happened to attend my college alumni meet-up; the theme of this meet-up was Giving Back. Until I was in the venue for this programme, I couldn't comprehend the exact meaning of this theme. There were students from different batches spanning over many years; the oldest of them were those who had passed out of college 50 years before me. I was overwhelmed with emotion. These old students, even though they had retired from their active life, yet they were actively participating in an event that I thought was more for the younger generations.

During my conversation with one such person, I understood the real reason they took so much effort to be there; they were there to help the younger generations not in terms of money but by giving back their decades of experience, which was priceless indeed. They were just going around mingling with fellow batch mates and giving out the lessons that none of the schools could teach. The best lessons that one can learn are the ones coming from another person's experience in life. It was a vivid recreation of the challenges they faced and how they overcame such obstacles in life. Even months of classroom sessions can't be compared to those live-sessions. I believe it is one of the key reasons why the world's top management schools get successful people from all over the world to reiterate their life lessons to their students. TED talks are an apt example. That reunion was one of my inspirations that pushed me to put my life lessons in this book.

I had suffered my part during my 20s and it took me a hard journey to gain back my health. This journey had taught me a few important lessons in terms of health. I realized most of my friends also had to go through similar hardships, and some still do, which can be dealt in a better way by understanding the key principles from the lessons I learned. I am not guaranteeing a complete cure to any physical illness but I am sure it can change the way people look at health and longevity.

As per the traditional medicines from ancient days, long before the birth of western medicine, there were 4448 identified diseases. With the constantly increasing population, diseases have also increased in parallel. Despite various developments in the field of medical sciences and technology, humanity is left with many challenging and life-threatening diseases such as cancer, cardiac diseases, metabolic disorders and virus outbreaks, which are yet to be solved. As the environment is getting more and more polluted, the available preventive measures for the diseases are to be valued better than the existing curative measures.

In the current decade alone, we have had some of the most threatening outbreaks (which include Ebola, Dengue, Swine Flu, Nipah, Influenza, Coronavirus, etc.) appearing all over the world. The amount of effort put in by the health organizations all over the world and each government to contain such outbreaks goes unnoticed when compared with the sensation created by the outbreak itself. Even though most of these outbreaks have been controlled, yet the time taken for this process of finding the right cure does take a toll on people and few of them don't survive the ordeal. The most common victims are elderly people and those with weak immune systems. Why now? Why not before?

Just decades ago, people were healthy with a strong immune system, which decreased the threat from these new types of outbreaks. Most of the people were able to sustain the impact of the various viral diseases and they survived without fear, which mitigated the threat factor. For instance, a person with a strong immune system can outsmart Swine flu without undergoing much of the sufferings. More than the actual virus, the one to look out for is one's fear and it should be treated as a serious concern. The most effective ways to prevent such outbreaks will be to improve the overall health and positive mindset of the common population across the world. The concepts discussed in this book will guide a person in this direction—basically, it means towards a healthy life.

Breath & BPM

The first and foremost phenomenon we need to understand is the breath we take in every moment. Yes! It is breath. I understand it's like telling an English teacher that the English language is made up of 26 alphabets. But I am sure your perception will change gradually as you go through the next few pages. So bear with me until you reach the end of this chapter to understand the importance of this concept.

Always start with basics first: what is breathing? Breathing means inhalation of oxygen from the air around us and exhalation of carbon dioxide that has accumulated inside our body. If you try to understand deeper, it means the process of taking in air is absorbing the oxygen and then expelling it is the release of carbon dioxide along with other gases that are not needed for the human body. The same can be explained in a few other ways in detail as well. The point is, a person is said to be living as long as he can breathe and will be declared dead the moment he stops taking a breath. And that is one of the reasons why it is an involuntary process in the human system.

Our body has a few involuntary processes and it's best if it's left alone. Does it mean that we shouldn't alter this process, or that we can't control this process? This question is best answered by Albert Einstein's quote:

"The definition of insanity is doing the same thing over and over again, but expecting different results."

So if you want better results, then you should try different methods. A word of caution though—if you wish to try different methods, you should have a good understanding of what you are trying to change. So before changing your breathing for better, you need to understand it.

Shallow Breathing

Normally what a human takes in what is called shallow breath. Shallow breathing or chest breathing means that a person takes in only the minimal quantity of air into his lungs wherein the number of breaths taken in a minute is usually 12 to 20. Calculating it for every minute, we end up expanding and contracting our lungs around 20 times approximately. This is normal for most of us. Nothing wrong about it but this number is a very important factor in deciding your longevity.

Deep Breathing

Deep breathing, on the other hand, means you take a good amount of air inside your lungs (as much as your lungs can hold). This usually takes a bit longer because of the efforts involved in expanding your chest to take in maximum and also exhale out the air again. There is no specific quantity that can be normalized as every person's lung capacity is different and the only common factor is the number of breaths a person takes within a minute. While practising deep breathing, the number of breaths per minute usually comes down to a number between six to nine, a significant 50% drop in the numbers when compared with the shallow breathing. This is the fact that you should remember before we proceed further.

BPM—Breath Per Minute

Now what makes the breath per minute (BPM) so important is that you use your muscles every time you perform breathing. Let's say you buy a new car with a pre-defined warranty in terms of maintenance-free time. For new cars, the average maintenance-free time or the effective running distance is around 150k to 200k kilometres, based on the build type, brand and usage. Likewise, our human body also comes with a warranty period, which has been mentioned in a few of the ancient medicinal studies books/manuscripts. So does it mean that if I bring down my BPM, it can increase my lifespan? Yes, provided you do it rightly. As mentioned in the first chapter, think of it as an addition and subtraction technique. You should know when to add and when to subtract otherwise your results will be wrong.

What happens when you try to hold your breath in an attempt to reduce your BPM while performing high-intensity workout? Most likely, you will faint due to lack of oxygen in your body. It might imply that those who don't do any workout can sustain for longer but that's wrong as well. If you don't give minimal movements to your muscles, gradually they will become stiff, which in turn will narrow your blood vessels. In the end, whatever fresh oxygen your nose gets into your lungs, it won't be reaching the muscles and organs, resulting in various illnesses. Exercise is important and also you can't reduce your BPM during workouts. We have 24 hours a day and throughout the period we do different sets of tasks. The list of tasks will vary from person to person except for a few standard ones like eating and sleeping. It is up to you to decide when to bring down your BPM because there is no single formula that can solve all problems. The key point is that you need to bring down your BPM count in a day. The breaths that you reduce are equal to ones you save for the future. This is similar to the money you save for the future.

Furthermore, keeping steady breathing is another principle that shouldn't be overlooked. I am sure you would have heard the proverb "Slow and steady wins the race." This brilliant proverb stands good for a lot of things in life and it holds perfect for breathing and longevity. With experience, I firmly believe that slowness and steadiness can win you any race. If you take life as a race, then slow and steady breathing will propel you towards longevity without a doubt. The fact is evident in a lot of scenarios—imagine you are driving the car at a 100 mph on a highway and suddenly an obstacle turns up over the corner. Unless you are a stunt driver, the first thing that happens when you see the obstacle is that you will go into a shock mode and your breathing becomes erratic. And assuming nothing bad happened, the most important thing that you will involuntarily work up is your breathing. If you have ever been in a shocking situation like that, you will know what I mean. Likewise, any severe medical condition will affect your breathing first, as it is one of the keys to reflect your physical condition. Medical practitioners very well understand this and that's why patients suffering from severe medical conditions are given an oxygen mask immediately.

And in any stressful scenario, the first response from your well-wisher will be to calm you down, which means you indirectly need to steady your breathing. You can try it anytime when you are in a stressful condition, just calm down your breathing and surprisingly you will recover from whatever it is that is disturbing you. No wonder most of the stress management techniques concentrate on your breathing.

Not just mental condition, any form of physical stress or a physical injury also causes unsteady breathing trying to bring a person down. If a person doesn't control his breathing within a particular time, he is bound to be unconscious because the oxygen supply to his brain will be disturbed and this causes your brain to go into a temporary shutdown. This is well understood by those who have engaged actively in sports. The first reaction of a coach when one of his trainees is injured is to make sure he gets some fresh air. The second will be to make sure his concentration doesn't divert and he or she is told to focus on the breathing side. Some people pass out even for a small physical injury, whereas some can keep their consciousness even after deep hit—the difference lies in how well the person has trained himself on his breathing techniques. Any other form of first aid is only secondary.

If steadying your breath can get you out of stressful conditions, why shouldn't we concentrate on that under normal circumstances? How you steady your breathing is up to you, there are many methods that you can follow. Almost all the wellness techniques start with breathing and there are many breathing techniques one can follow based on the condition. I follow meditation and pranayama to keep my breathing steady but I will leave that research to you as long as you understand the importance of steady breathing.

Deep Breathing

Until now, we have seen two important techniques—reduce your BPM and steady your breathing. The third technique is deep breathing: if you practice all the three techniques correctly, it will eventually lead you to the ultimate goal of good health. They might all look trivial and the same but it is better if you understand the importance and difference between each of them in detail. For this, one needs to master all three of them.

In an article about cancer, Dr. Otto Warburg, 1931 Noble Prize winner, has indicated that oxygen as the deadliest enemy of cancer. He has also emphasized the importance of deep breathing. Not just cancer, most of our ailments can be handled by controlling the amount of air we breathe in. The one who maximizes his breath intake will have a better functioning body. This is a well-established rule among monks, martial artists, yoga practitioners, sportspeople and other high-performance individuals. This is quite remarkable because most of the top performers do it with deep breathing. But in reality, the process doesn't involve any special skill and none of our breaths can absorb any special ingredient from the air. It's the same air that everybody breathes in but the difference is only the quantity of air. How is that possible?

Consider a motorbike with a fuel tank capacity of 10 litres. If the person fills the tank with 10 litres, the bike can cover 100 miles, whereas if he fills only nine litres the same bike can run only for 90 miles. This difference of 10 miles is the difference between those who do deep breathing versus those who do shallow breathing. The below table will make it more clear.

Breath Intake Capacity	Individuals
> 80%	High energy levels, strong immunity
> 50%	Normal energy levels, susceptible to external infections
< 50%	Reduced energy levels, reduced organ functions leading to sickness and suffering

You have to formulate your schedule, as no one knows you better than yourself. Bringing down your BPM every hour is not a practical one unless you are one of those privileged ones who spend your whole day in an ashram or secluded spot with all the basic amenities at your arm's reach.

"Breath is like your money, use it wisely and you will achieve prime health. Breath is Wealth."

If health is wealth, then breath also can be accumulated like wealth.

Wealth	Breath
Reduce your expenses and save for future	Reduce your BPM and save it for future
Have a steady income	Follow a steady breathing habit
Bigger the investment, bigger the returns	Deeper your breath, better your health

Animal BPM and Longevity

We will look at a few facts about other animals with which we share this common concept. You can observe the animal kingdom for more examples. In the "Tortoise and the Rabbit Race" story, the tortoise has an average lifespan of 80 to 120 years whereas a rabbit lives for only 1–2 years. The reason behind this is quite evident—the tortoise's BPM (3–4) is much slower than that of the rabbit's BPM (30–60). Similarly, you can look at different mammals and their corresponding lifespan from the few examples listed below.

Mammal	BPM	Avg. lifespan (in Yrs)
Dog	24	10–13
Cat	20–30	2–6
Horse	12	25–30
Cheetah	60	10–12
Elephant	10–12	70–80

There are some interesting observations here, the BPM of a horse and an elephant are close to each other but there is a considerable difference in their average lifespan. I attribute the difference to two important factors. One is the capacity of air they breathe in every time; second, the BPM of a horse can reach up to 150 while running, whereas the elephant hardly runs. Nevertheless, the importance of BPM and the capacity of the air we humans take in play a very important role in deciding our longevity, which is very much evident from the above examples.

O$_2$ Clinics

One of the recent developments in healing forms is the use of oxygen overdose for a specific timeframe, which helps in overall healing and also improves bodily functions. These clinics make you inhale pure oxygen for a specific amount of time and that does all the magic. Of course, you will need to pay for it. You may reason out that we are surrounded by oxygen also, but, unfortunately, our hazardous advancements in various fields have polluted our Mother Nature to the extent that we are forced to go for treatments like this. With the present conditions, the O$_2$ clinics are a better choice when you decide to take up natural healing path. Hopefully, the awareness to breathe fresh air and its subsequent benefits are taken seriously by people and they can find a way to reverse these conditions. Until then, that would mean being constantly aware of your environment and the way you breathe. The easier alternative will be to visit a virgin getaway location once in a while to enjoy pollution free air. Even a friend of mine joked about a new business venture to provide people with fresh air in the form of a container to breathe, just like a water bottle. It might sound childish but I wouldn't be surprised if it becomes a reality tomorrow.

Takeaways

- Steady Breathing

- Reduce BPM

- Deep Breathing

In summary, most of the important body functions are controlled by the air in our system. Key ones include heartbeat, eyelash movement and excretion of waste. If there is an imbalance of air in our body, all of these important involuntary functions will be affected, causing various sickness and in some cases fatal conditions. Hence, one needs to keep a balance on this air element and this can be achieved by the three techniques we have discussed in the above sections. And before we end this chapter, breathing techniques need not be limited to the concepts discussed here; there are various other good concepts that have been studied and preached by masters, which can be availed from the right sources.

Elixir of Life

During my primary school days, nearly 20 years back, we had a chapter on water in my science syllabus. Water was symbolized as the Elixir of Life, but during those days, I didn't realize the importance of it. All that I can remember from that chapter is that the questions were quite easy because they just talked about water and we didn't have to memorize formulas or numeric values; eventually it became one of my most memorable chapters. In recent times, after my involvement in different studies on the alternative medicine field, I am amazed at the relevance of water in our contemporary life. After breathing, the next important thing a human needs for survival is water. Humans can survive for weeks with just water and no intake of solid food; on the other hand, an average human cannot survive for more than four days without water. Water is such an important part of our life, not only in our day-to-day survival but also by playing a vital role in expanding our lifespan and maintaining our wellbeing.

Our human body is made out of 70% water and it is necessary to make sure our body remains hydrated at all costs. Water helps us in a lot of ways; few of the key ones include regulating body temperature, toxin removal, improve mobility, etc. Since this is one of the most important factors for our survival, each one of us has been gifted with what I like to call our internal "water manager." This water manager doesn't need external guidance and this guy can tell you all about your body's water needs. He is the one who tells you when your body needs water in the form of thirst. But over time, we have outlearnt ourselves to forget the triggers that are being sent by our body. External conditions like air-conditioned rooms, etc. have only covered up our natural reflexes to indicate and warn.

"Drink when you are thirsty is the past; make sure you are thirsty is our future."

This is a very important point, which needs to be understood. For example, when only fans were available, our internal water manager was working fine and there were constant reminders of our water needs. We rarely realized the goodness of water and we never appreciated our internal water manager. We stayed healthier without the need to worry over sickness. But after the invention of fully air-conditioned buildings (including both homes and workplaces), we seldom feel our water needs because we seldom do any strenuous task. So we rarely feel thirsty and we tend to drink very little water throughout our day. We become waterless zombies spending two-third of a day in office spaces and the other one-third in our homes sitting in front of air conditioners. As a result, we invite all possible forms of sickness that can arise due to water imbalance in our body.

So the ground rule for the current generation is that you need to keep reminders to remind yourselves of your water needs and stay hydrated. See how funny it sounds and yet how serious it is. This is the beauty of our present lifestyle, we have developed from a point where we didn't need efforts to remember our water needs to a point we need to put in additional efforts to remind our self of our own needs. The irony is that we call this process as technological advancement and sophisticated life.

For instance, whenever a person falls sick, the best advice for the patient will be to take water-rich foods, which include juices, fresh fruits, porridge and other similar items. This is because indirectly we are reassuring our water balance so that our body can do its normal functions without fail.

Eat Your Water

This is another underlying principle, which needs to be kept in mind. I am sure you would have heard this famous phrase from many health experts but the real question is how many of you follow it? 'Eat your water' simply means take it slow. Like our discussion in the last chapter regarding the breathing and the benefits of breathing slowly, the same can be applied to water as well. Let's say you have an iron rod heated red and suddenly you pour water on it. What happens? When you gulp water immediately after a workout or a strenuous activity, a similar reaction will happen inside your body. Again taking cold water is the opposite of what we just saw, our body maintains an optimum temperature to keep us alive and whenever you gulp cold water this fire inside us will be disturbed causing health issues. So the reason why experts tell you to eat your water is to make sure you adjust the water to suit your body temperature and slowly take it in. Yes, that's the secret behind 'eating your water.' When you take a mouthful of water and hold it in your mouth, two things happen.

- The water gets adjusted to your body temperature.

- The water gets mixed with enough saliva to make it ideal for absorption.

So remember even though it has been told several times I would still reiterate, the best way is to take water in is to eat it.

How Do You Maintain a Fish Tank?

One can learn a lot from the art of maintaining a simple fish tank in our house. There are varieties of fish tanks. Irrespective of the variations, the ground rule to keep your fish alive is to have a clean environment for the fish to strive. For example, you can install oxygen blower to increase the quality of water, then a temperature controller to maintain the optimum temperature for the fish, then an automated cleaning mechanism, or use a specific breed of fish to clean the tank. Having all these sophistications still doesn't rule out the process of cleaning the fish tank regularly. Maybe the tanks with such sophistication don't need to be cleaned, as frequently as a normal one but at the end of the day, this super sophisticated fish tank also needs cleaning. Cleaning here means changing the water inside the tank and washing off the container itself. Now, what correlation does this have with our topic here?

I believe some of you would have already made the relation; our body is like the fish tank and our blood is the water in the tank. Everyone knows that kidneys do the most cleaning up of our body that includes blood, but for the kidney to function properly, it needs enough water. The kidney eliminates toxins through sweat, urine and faeces. In this phenomenon, the kidney invariably depletes our body's water content and we need a good amount of water intake to counter this water loss and make this process more efficient. So the next time you see a fish tank, whether a clean one or a dirty one, remember this correlation and drink enough water.

Let the Water Flow

To make it easier to understand the importance of water further, let's take the example of a water tunnel.

A water tunnel might have stones, curves and other obstacles that block the flow of water. These blockages result in the accumulation of wastes in and around the blockages. This is because the water flow is not sufficient enough to carry away the impurities. When these canals are filled with water, these accumulated waste materials get washed away. Likewise, our body is a set of closed tunnels with a lot of curves, twists and blockages. So we must keep our water flow within our body at optimum levels, which signifies the importance of maintaining the water content in our body. If you don't, then your body will slowly become a warehouse of toxins that get accumulated over a period and it can cause you all types of illness. So make sure that the water flow is constant always and you don't have to worry about toxins or any other related conditions.

The above few examples are just a reminder for you to understand the importance of water intake and you don't need high-level research materials to prove this simple fact. It is simply logical to understand this process. I hope you take water a little more seriously from now, especially if you are serious about longevity.

Takeaways

- Eat your Water
- Maintain your Fish Tank

Food

In this chapter, we will be looking at the basics of the relationship between food, health and longevity. Food is anything that you take in; it gives us the energy to do everything in day-to-day life. The quantity of food intake depends on several factors; some of the key ones include age, gender, individual physiology, nature of work, habits, emotional state, economic conditions, taste preferences, etc. Irrespective of everything, food is our fuel and it is similar to an automotive engine, which needs petrol or diesel for their functioning. We won't be going into details of the food mechanism; rather, we will be looking at the theory of two important processes in our food cycle with a more simplified example. The first part is the digestive mechanism. Digestion decides how much we get out of our food intake and how healthy we become after every meal. The second one is the excretion mechanism, which removes the unwanted things from our body; in other words, we can call them the toxin removal process. Both these processes are intrinsically related and play a very important role in deciding our health as well as lifespan.

Become a Master Chef

I am not sure how many of you reading this book is a real chef, but based on my experience mastery of culinary art is not limited to only professional chefs alone rather even most low-income class have a fair experience at being a chef. My all-time favourite chef, of course, is my mom. The reason why I brought in the culinary art here is not to define recipes for health and longevity but to explain the basics of culinary art and its relationship with longevity. I too indulge in cooking whenever time permits and it is a stress buster for me. My cooking experience dates back to my younger days. I started cooking when I was 12 years old, and this habit has led me to understand the relation between the process of digestion and cooking. So I will be explaining the digestion part from a culinary point of view. I believe it makes it much simpler to understand when you relate a few things.

On the contrary to the normal belief that digestion starts from the stomach, it starts from your mouth. The moment our saliva gets mixed with food digestion starts and then later, the process continues in the stomach. Now consider the stomach as a closed cooking pot. The first process in cooking starts with getting the necessary ingredients followed by heating the cooking vessel with a fire source. Then comes adding in the right ingredients, at the right interval, in the right quantity, at the right moment. Then you wait and give time for the food to be cooked. The factor that differentiates a great cook and an ordinary one is the mastery of the above-mentioned activities. A simple flaw in the measurement of the ingredients or a slightly hurried process can transform a signature dish into an unpleasant experience for the palate. Likewise mastering our digestive mechanism basics will significantly improve your health. There are a few differences here between our stomach and a normal cooking pot.

Always Burning Cooking Pot

Unlike the gas burner used for cooking, the heat source in our body never turns off; in other words, the stomach is always under the heat source. This is quite needed because as per traditional beliefs the moment the heat source turns off, we die. (It is evident from the fact that the moment a person dies his body becomes colder as time passes by.) So if our stomach is always under a heat source, then you can imagine what will happen if its left ideal without anything to cook, but the good part is that it is our own fire source working under a controlled environment and the intensity of heat is reasonable to the extent of our human body can tolerate. Sometimes, we tend to trip off beyond this limit and so the stomach walls get damaged.

To avoid such conditions, we should make sure there is something for our pot (stomach) to cook at all times. Usually, we can confirm if a normal cooking vessel is heated to the right extent by feeling the heat slightly above the cooking pot but we don't have the luxury to do the same thing with our stomach. But our body has its way of telling us when the pot is heated and ready for food—this trigger is called hunger.

When you ignore this trigger, eventually, you will damage the stomach walls and develop conditions leading to ailments like acidity, ulcer and similar conditions. And once your cooking pot (stomach) is damaged, then it will directly affect your quality of health and in turn your longevity. Now, can you see the correlation between a normal cooking pot and our stomach?

The next step is to identify the right ingredients— in our case, it means the quality of food. The better the quality of food, the better your health becomes. I won't be explaining much on this point because this is the common focal point of numerous books and there are several experts who can advise on this as well.

The final part of cooking is patience. Let's say you take out a dish from the vessel before it is fully cooked or you add in some ingredients at the wrong moment. It will turn out to be a bad recipe. The same applies to our digestive system as well. Eat only when you are hungry; if sometimes you don't have this trigger, it means your body is still processing the last meal. You need to give your body enough time to finish digesting the previous meal. So it is nothing wrong to skip a meal if you don't feel hunger.

Cooking	Digestion
Identify the right ingredients	Quality of food consumed
Wait for the cooking pot to reach the ideal temperature	Eat when you get the hunger trigger
Be patient till the cooking completes	Skip the meal if you aren't hungry

Closed Barbeque Pot

Similar to the above metaphor, our stomach can also be compared to a closed barbeque vessel that requires a few precautions and additional procedures to be followed. The most common issue with closed barbeque setup is that the inner part of the meat sometimes may not be cooked properly. If you increase the heat to counter this problem, then the outer layer will get burnt quickly. It's all about finding the optimal conditions to cook the whole meat properly or the whole dish cooked to perfection. For instance, when cooking meat, the usual way will be to cut the meat into smaller pieces so that the heat spreads equally and it is well cooked.

Barbecuing also calls for the process of marinating the meat or other vegetables. Usually, the cleaned ingredients are mixed with the right set of spices, mixed well and left ideal for a few minutes so that the spices can be absorbed into the meat and vegetables. This process significantly enhances the quality of the final cooked dish. How do we marinate food, which is already cooked and ready to be consumed? In the body, when the food is taken into the mouth, we need to mix it with enough saliva and chew it properly so that when the food reaches your stomach, it is ready for digestion. Usually, we tend to limit the chewing part to two or three times and just swallow our food, thereby overloading our stomach's process. This needs to be avoided as a rule. The corollary of "Eat your Water" therefore is "Drink your Food." Drink your food signifies two important processes.

1. Chewing your food properly and making sure that there are no big pieces and eases the digestion process.

2. The more time you chew, the more saliva gets mixed with your food and saliva is one of the key ingredients for the digestion process.

Barbeque	Digestion
Marinate	Mix your food with saliva in your mouth
Break larger pieces of meat into small ones to ease cooking	Chew properly to break solid food into liquid form to ease digestion

Key Points to Note

- Value the importance of Body triggers (Hunger)

- Drink your Food

Eat with your Senses

There are several ways to interpret this statement but as far as this book is concerned, it is to interpret in the below two ways.

1. First, eat with your five senses.

2. Secondly, eat with timing sense.

Let's look at each of the above with examples. (Examples help us remember better, especially if you are like me with limited memory.)

Firstly, the five senses are sight, smell, hearing, touch and taste. These five senses are needed to eat and enjoy any kind of food. That is, every time you want to eat, make sure you

- See (the food)

- Smell (its flavour)

- Hear (say the name of the dish aloud)

- Feel (it with your fingers)

- Taste (it in your tongue before swallowing it)

It might look trivial at this moment but look at your eating habits and honestly, I believe a very few of us do this.

Secondly, eat with timing sense, which is eating at the right intervals. Make sure you do justice to the name 'breakfast'—break the fast—it signifies the activity of breaking the night long fast by a person in the next day morning. Similarly, lunch at noon and dinner in the evenings is the right way to have it. As the famous adage goes:

"Have breakfast like a king, lunch like a prince and dinner like a pauper."

Let us look at a scenario for you to understand the two principles beyond doubt. Assuming you have a house party and invited ten people for lunch, to guarantee the success of the party I am sure you will be performing all the below activities.

Lunch party	Every meal timing
You will be fixing an appropriate date and time and will proceed to invite the guests a little earlier so that they fix their schedule to be at your house on the said day at the said time.	This is synonymous with fixing your time for every meal.

On the day of the event, you would be calling them up with a reminder note to confirm their presence and also would request them for food restrictions they might have. After hearing their answers, you will convey it to your cooks so they prepare a delicious meal to delight your guests.	This is synonymous to hearing the name of your everyday meal. You are informing your digestive system to be ready for what's coming in.
The next thing will be for you to display the spread of food items with the smell of its wonderful flavours filling the whole house. This is to appease the guests with varieties of food and their delicious smell.	This is synonymous to seeing the food and smelling the flavours in it. This is a confirmation to your digestive system to prepare itself for the incoming meal.
Additionally, to make it look special, you may opt to serve your guests all by yourself.	This is synonymous to you using your own hands or fingers to eat your meal. It is the final verification by the digestive system.
Your guests get to enjoy the meal and I am sure they will remember the experience for life.	You achieve prime health and longevity.

If you can do so much for your guest, why not do better for yourself? I know it might not be practical to follow all these points for every meal, but it's your health and lifespan we are talking about, so make it a point to follow at least a few of them on possible occasions. The toughest one I believe will be the use of own fingers because, in this generation spoons, forks, knives, chopsticks have taken precedence over our fingers.

This can be attributed to the evolution of humankind. Our Western ancestors needed knives and sharp tools alike to eat raw meat. When better cooking methods developed and dining became sophisticated spoons, forks, knives became more common. While our Eastern ancestors used different kinds of roots and small tree branches to eat food to avail their medical benefits; later on these evolved into chopsticks with no medical benefits. The middle-Asian countries still predominantly eat with their hands and fingers as grains and millets form a major portion of their food. Having said all this, there is always a gap between the ideal way and practical way. So I will leave the decision to you when it comes to following either of this one.

Taste the Flavours of Life

"If you don't taste the flavours of the food you can't feel the flavours of life."

The other most commonly overlooked fact is the benefits of having all the six tastes in a meal. Irrespective of the cultural differences there is one underlying principle among the food traditions in our older generations. There will at least be one food item to satisfy all our different taste buds. The reason has deep roots in medical science. Over time this has been overlooked, resulting in people becoming susceptible to different forms of ailments. If you look at each of the different tastes, it has its own significance in maintaining our health conditions. You may refer to the below table for the explanation. I have quoted the below from one of my medical study material to imply the underlying importance.

Taste	Benefits	Stimulates & Strengthens
Bitter	Excellent germicide against harmful bacteria inside the stomach and intestines increases resistance to poisons and toxins	Heart, Small Intestine
Salty	Reduces muscle cramps, improves memory power, cools down the body	Kidneys and bladder
Pungent (Hot)	Warms up the body, flushes out toxins	Lungs, colon and blood circulation
Astringent	Blood clotting	Nervous system
Sweet	Builds bodily tissues, provides energy	Blood circulation

Continued...

Sour	Purifies blood vessels, provides instant energy and helps in the absorption of nutrients in food	Liver and gall bladder

Even though there are quite a few examples that can be quoted to support the above table, the use of lemon and salt is the best. During my childhood, whenever we used to go for a basketball tournament, our coach would bring along a few lemons and a small salt packet. During the short breaks between the sessions, he would slice the lemons, apply salt on it and would advise us to consume the juice drops from it. I never realized the actual use of it until recently. The sour taste helps in instant energy, improves nutrient absorption from the last eaten meal and the salt reduces muscle cramps, regulates the body temperature and the kidneys, as we sweat a lot. But now the market is filled with a lot of isotonic drinks, which indirectly have the same benefits of consuming lemon and salt and this simple habit is being forgotten. It is, of course, will always be part of my childhood memories.

Certain people are habituated to only a particular taste or in certain cases they prefer a blunt taste wherein the flavours are not felt properly. This habit needs a slight tweak. Food does have an impact on our emotions as well. This is basic science. Our psychological emotions are a result of various chemicals and food itself is a set of chemical substances. So if you follow a food style or follow a similar food habit always, it means you will have the same set of emotions, which will pave the way for dullness in your lifestyle. I do understand it is good to have a stable lifestyle with the same routine throughout but if there are no momentary ups and downs, then life will become a bore. This boredom at the beginning might look insignificant but if it is allowed to dwell over for some time, then they become toxic similar to a perishable food item. Boredom can drive you into the negative side, which is quite tough to rectify later on.

Taste has proved to have an impact on our mood and this has led people to use tastes as a metaphor to describe their feelings. This opens up a new dimension on foods but I would leave it your sole discretion to pursue it further. Some of the examples to trigger your thought are as below.

"Sweet as sugar."

"It was a bitter experience."

"He was hot as chillies."

"He was sour from a day-long journey."

Takeaways

- Become a master chef

- Eat with your senses

- Drink your food

- Taste the flavours of life

Irreplaceable Doctors

There are several general medical consultants and specialists to address different kinds of health conditions. Based on the economic conditions and locality of the people, they get to access one of the facilities. The most important factor will be the financial condition of the patient. In recent times, you can't survive a medical condition without a medical insurance card. The medical bill can easily create a black hole in your pocket. (And if the disease doesn't kill you the medical bill will!)

Under these circumstances, what if I tell you there are three doctors available to you at your doorstep and they never charge any fees to help you? Yes, I know it sounds like a dream but it is true and has been proved several times under different studies. These three doctors have always been with us and healing us from the time humans walked on earth. Our ancestors appreciated this fact and took full advantage of this luxury. However, the later generations have forgotten these doctors and their powerful healing techniques. One piece of interesting information

I perceive from our history is that in previous centuries the doctor's status and his skills were decided by the type of disease he could cure. If a doctor could cure fatal conditions he was considered as the best in the field, whereas, unfortunately, in recent days, the best doctors are decided by the fees they charge for treating a condition. I won't say it is wrong because the way of living has evolved over the recent decades and especially without money it would be a different scenario. Naturally, an advanced diagnosis has been made possible by the latest inventions, which takes time, efforts and investments, which is why the cost of medication has significantly increased in recent times.

"Prevention is better than cure."

This proverb is the first one that comes to most people's minds when illness and medicines are being discussed. This fact is proved over and over again. If you want to achieve longevity, this should be your chant. Let me put this in a simpler form, assuming your car had a malfunction with one of its working parts and it needs to be changed. You can take it to the best mechanic to fix it and get the part replaced with the original spare part but still, it is considered lesser than a new one. Our human body is similar to this car, repaired but not perfect.

At this juncture, we should acknowledge the fact that everyone will fall sick from time-to-time.

Falling sick is normal for any human being, but the important point is recovering from the illness without having any other consequences, or side effects. The three doctors we are going to see in this chapter are experts in this and there is no equal for them in keeping us safe from illness or in other words preventing illness. The more you stay in unison with them, the higher are your chances of staying away from sickness or any other medical conditions. I believe there is no equal for a mom's affection and love, but not all of us are privileged enough to have a mom living with us all the time. But the mother I am referring to here is our Mother Nature. She, on the other hand, is always there.

Universal Mother

"Planet Earth is the only known planet among the nine others in our solar system that supports life."

The importance of this statement is forgotten most of the time. If every individual understands and values this point, then the quality of life on this planet will be much better. I would prefer calling Mother Nature instead of Planet Earth because it has a personal touch when the word mother gets included.

Firstly, human life was made possible by this diversified ecosystem, which includes the availability of water, optimum climate, gravity and other key factors that are available only on this planet.

When Mother Nature can create life, she can protect life as well. Protection from ailments is what I mean. We humans have evolved and have improved our life to an extent where we can identify and treat most of our ailments and also extend this to other animals to a certain extent. In this book, however, we will stick to humans only.

For humans, all these improvements have been made possible only in the last few centuries but life has been flourishing on this planet for a very long time. How was it possible then? Our Mother Nature has protected us in her own way. Most of us have been blind to this side of Mother Nature. We can even say we have not spent enough effort to value it until recently. With the growing awareness in improving the quality of human life, most of the researches are aimed in this direction and most of them have started understanding this rule. The more we connect with Mother Nature, the better are our chances of staying healthy.

Connect with Mother Nature

Our universal mother is so nice that all we have to do is just connect with her and she will reward you with all the goodness. Just like charging your phone or any other device, all that you need to do is connect. There are several ways to do it. I will give a few simple and most effective ways that have already been proved by various researches.

Barefoot Walk

In the past, almost everyone spent enough time walking barefoot every day. This has been the practice because in those days slippers and shoes were considered a luxury item. Later on, it became a necessity and nowadays more so of a fashion statement. I understand you need protection for your foot but that shouldn't restrict you from walking barefoot at least a few times in a day. In parts of the world where living is still not modernized, people walk barefoot most of the time and it never bothers them, even protection is never a concern. If you look closely, their health is much better than their counterparts.

Why?

Is it possible?

Just walking with barefoot can heal ailments?

The answers to these questions are being researched and new interesting answers turn up every day. One of the answers that I feel is more convincing scientifically is that our Mother Nature is the storehouse of positive ions and she discharges these positive ions to those who wish to receive it. When you walk barefoot, you directly connect with this positive ion warehouse and your body gets charged up. They reduce inflammations, thereby reducing pain and bestowing other benefits.

Additionally, it is a well-established fact that the pressure points in our foot are very effective and just by activating these points, our bodily functions can return to normal. There are foot massage techniques that are used to heal various ailments. Walking barefoot does the same activation of the points on the foot. How different can it be when pressure is applied to a point by a person and when the same pressure is applied by our weight? The only notable difference will be that for getting someone to massage your foot, you need to spend money whereas for walking barefoot you need to spend your energy (in other words burn some calories). Wonderful, isn't it?

There are no hard and fast rules for walking barefoot—just remove your footwear and start walking. As long as the terrain is manageable, you can start doing it anywhere. The effects are quite visible within just seven days. I walk barefoot whenever when I go for a walk with my dog, based on the advice from my teacher, who is a medical practitioner in traditional medicine. The benefits I have received have been tremendous. Moreover, intrigued by this activity, one of my neighbours started following it too. In just a week, he visited me personally and thanked me as this single activity had helped him with his chronic hip and knee pain.

Bring Nature Indoors

In the olden days, people used to live in houses made of wood and mud structures. But with the invention of cement, we have moved on to build cemented houses, which are very much necessary for a safe living. One thing to remember though is that these cement walls insulate you from both harmful things and also good things. This reduces our connectivity with Mother Nature. So to achieve safety and also health benefits, we need antennas to boost connectivity. If your radio connectivity is not strong enough, then we install antennas inside our houses to increase the range. Similarly, we need antennas too to connect with Mother Nature. Indoor plants are the antennas inside the house to increase the signal connectivity with Mother Nature. Having indoor plants inside the house improves the air quality, removes toxins in the air, reduces stress and improves the quality of sleep. All these relate to health.

Other than indoor plants, having a water system inside the house also helps. The water system doesn't mean letting the water flow through your living room and bedrooms; I am talking about a controlled water system, which could be a water fountain or a small indoor pond. Keeping a water system inside the house also regulates the indoor temperature and the vaporized water particles combine with the harmful foreign elements in the air dragging them down.

Due to this process, the foreign particles are dragged down with weight and eventually, the air gets purified. For instance, in Kuala Lumpur yearly once there's this haze phenomenon. The air quality index usually sores to unhealthy levels sometimes even to hazardous levels in certain places. This is a result of the smoke emitted by burning forests in certain countries, which is being blown over to the neighbouring countries by the sea currents. Usually, this haze stays as a guest in Malaysia for a period varying from three to five weeks and during this time the most effective ways to keep your indoor atmosphere healthy is by having indoor plants and also a water system.

In a nutshell, by bringing nature indoors, you connect with nature and simultaneously improve your quality of life. This is one of the key factors that can have a good effect on your overall health and longevity.

Vacation and Getaways

Sometimes you have to reach out to Mother Nature. It's like paying a visit to your friend, the more often you visit, the stronger the bond becomes. It's similar to any human relationship, the more time you spend on a relationship, the stronger it becomes. Eventually, when you reach out to Mother Nature more often, she showers you with remarkable benefits. And the most interesting part is it's cheap and more beneficial when compared to other human relationships.

Vacation

Vacations can be the much-needed relief for all busy people running on their toes throughout the day. Even the most accomplished person will earn a vacation once in a while. They are the number one stress busters. If you look closely, some key points have been explained below.

Getaways

Getaways are the recent remedy to all people suffering from stress. Especially, in recent years getaways are becoming more and more popular. The reason behind this is the feel-good benefits you receive when you go on a vacation. And if you look closely, the getaway locations are mostly picked based on this connect with nature concept. Will you consider a vacation at a bustling city as a getaway? Irrespective of what that city can showcase, the manmade ventures are no match for the natural ones. Just a relaxed evening on the beach, a morning stroll through a virgin forest, a relaxing view of the sunshine over the hill can heal you to an immeasurable extent.

Hiking

Hiking is one of the activities in which your physical exertion doesn't bother you much. That's because of the feel-good factors you get while hiking. To realize this benefit, all you need to do is just imagine walking through an unmarked terrain with a group of friends and you will feel refreshed. Imagine then the experience of a real hike! In developed and developing countries, these nature sports are becoming more and more popular because of this point.

Forest Bathing or Shinrin-yoku

This is a Japanese concept, which also emphasizes the importance of connecting with nature. *Shinrin* in Japanese means forest and *yoku* means bath. Forest bathing means bathing in a forest atmosphere or absorbing nature through your senses. This technique emphasizes the concept of being in unison with nature to receive amazing benefits. It is simply being in nature, connecting with it through our senses of sight, hearing, taste, smell and touch. This activity has proved to improve your mood, relax and rejuvenate you. To know more about this intriguing concept, you may consider reading *Forest Bathing: How Trees Can Help You Find Health and Happiness* by Dr. Qing Li.

Immerse in Ocean

Yes. The ocean is another source of positive energy. If you have had a chance to learn any of the energy healing techniques like Reiki healing or Pranic healing or similar ones, you will appreciate the importance of saltwater. In all these methods, they use saline water to cleanse the negativity in our system and its surroundings. It is even suggested to bath in saline water to remove all the negative energy around your aura. Maybe it looks spiritual but if you understand the scientific explanation, one of the key benefits of saline water is that it is a disinfectant and protects against a variety of bacteria. Miraculously, our Mother Nature has provided us with such vast oceans but we seldom acknowledge or reap benefit from it. Just a simple bath from the ocean or a walk on the beach with the waves washing against your feet will give a soothing feeling. No wonder crowds throng the beaches in the mornings and evenings, whether they actually understand the benefits they are reaping or not. Maybe not everyone will have easy access to the ocean or sea; in that case, you should make it a point to choose a sea-getaway for your holidays.

If the ocean is not accessible, a simple dive into a nearby pool can give you the same relaxation. Pool exercises are by far the most sought after recovery method, especially after a heavy workout. Almost all the sports athletes are advised to go swimming after their training. This is because scientifically swimming has proven to boost the body's recovery quickly. In recent times, most apartment complexes come with a swimming pool and yet people hardly realize the importance of swimming and make use of the facilities. Only a meagre number of people accounting for < 5% of a community uses the swimming pool. In my personal experience too I have had wonderful recovery after a dip in the pool, especially after running my marathons. I find it the best way to recover, which can revitalize my body with enough water content and bring down my body's temperature to an optimal range. The healing nature is in the water element, which in itself is an integral part of our Mother Nature. From now on every time you pass through a swimming pool, I urge you to think about the importance and the effectiveness of swimming.

If you co-relate all the above points, you will understand the reason why all the exotic tourist destinations have one or more of this nature's touch. The health benefits and the effect of such touch on our minds are far beyond explanation. Most of the upcoming community designs, almost 90% of them, include nature's touch in their plan. They have water bodies, a park, a walking area, swimming pools, ample sunlight conditions and indoor and outdoor plants. These are the current USPs for all real estate people. The most luxurious mansions owned by celebrities and the wealthy may even have a mini forest in their surroundings.

In summary, there are a few methods based on their acceptance, have been made popular to the entire world population and there could be few more localized versions of this concept of connecting with nature. I will leave that point for you to synergize your nearest option. Thus goes the relationship between health and Mother Nature. The important lesson to be learned irrespective of the type of the method followed are the benefits one receives by connecting with nature. It all concludes at one point.

"Connecting with nature significantly improves your chances of health and long life."

Indomitable Sun

The sun, the ultimate source of light to the world, is another irreplaceable healing energy. Without the sun, there would be no life possible on this planet. From the time of our ancestors, the sun has been worshipped as a god. They had their reasons to pronounce so but the underlying importance can't be denied even in this technologically advanced era. The practice of praying to the sun has been in existence in all ancient cultures. We can find many references, including Hindu mythology. Today this practice has been researched at an extensive level. The research is still going on but what has been established as a concrete fact is that our human body should be exposed to the sun for a minimum extent of time every day.

For an average human being, the exposure to the sun should be at least 30 minutes every day. These 30 minutes of exposure to the sun can provide us with Vitamin D that is much needed for the strengthening of our bones, teeth, immune system, brain and nervous systems. There are a few more benefits that can be added to this list. If we cannot get exposed to the recommended 30 minutes of sunlight, then we need to include a good quantity of food supplements to replenish Vitamin D. Our body needs different kinds of nutrients daily. Ideally, no one can get the right amount of nutrients in their daily intake every day due to various factors. That's the reason why we reach out for supplements. Now, if you want to supplement Vitamin D, which is available in abundance in nature, absolutely free of cost, with something costlier, is that really smart? Even if you are super rich and you can afford to buy anything, if you are substituting a part of your meal to Vitamin D eventually, you will miss out on some other nutrient that can be supplemented only through your food intake. It is similar to accumulating wealth; you should always be looking at versatile sources to be successful. So the next time you get a chance to walk in the sun, do enjoy the heat and warmth because you are doing yourself a favour being in the sunlight.

There is an interesting concept called 'sun gazing'—it is the act of looking directly at the sun during dawn and dusk. This concept has been in existence since the 1960s and only recently, its beneficial effects are being debated and researched over. Most of the scientists state that looking into the sun might cause medical conditions but there are a few who have proved them wrong by adopting this process. Some of the benefits include increased energy levels, vitality, eyesight improvement, increase in pineal gland size, improvement in psychic attributes and overall health. Even during World War I, doctors exposed the wounded soldiers to sunlight due to its healing effects. In a testimonial from a Korean War veteran, it is mentioned that when he was held as a prisoner during wartime, he was forced to stare at the sun along with few more war prisoners for 10 hours a day continuously without looking aside or closing their eyes. This was supposed to be a punishment but what happened surprised everyone. He, along with other prisoners, instead, reaped positive benefits from this punishment. Those who wore glasses to supplement their eyesight no longer needed them because the daily sunlight exposure drastically improved their eyesight and also their overall health. Even in his seventies, this person has confirmed he didn't need glasses.

The same sun gazing is practised by the Westerners in a slightly different way called sunbathing, where they expose their bare skin to sunlight to improve their skin and compensate all the Vitamin D that they have lost. They get themselves tanned in this process but they don't directly look into the sunlight with their eyes. Nevertheless, there are benefits for this process without which a whole lot of people wouldn't be following it for so long a period. Likewise, the benefits of being in sunlight during dawn and dusk are already proved beneficial beyond doubts.

Having said all these I wouldn't suggest you go out to start staring at the sun throughout the day at one shot, firstly it is not practical and the beneficial effects of sun gazing are still in the early research stages only. However, the underlying point is to appreciate the beneficial effects of the sun and to understand the importance of exposing oneself to the sun for a few minutes every day. I hope this section influences your bias about sunlight and exposure to it.

Your Partner for Life!

Without a second thought, I can tell that everyone is gifted with a partner who never leaves you whatever may be the situation. As long as you take care of this partner of yours there is no force in the world, which can put you down, the sad part is that most of the people never acknowledge this partner and end with all the forms of troubles. As long as this partner believes in you, you can achieve whatever you want. Your best chance against any form of sickness, either physical or mental, is this partner. I am sure most of you will be curious to know this partner. It's none other than your own body. Let me say it again

> **"Your body is your partner for life."**

Our immune system is the strongest weapon or medicine against any form of illness. All the medicines and treatment that we avail is just to boost our immune system directly or indirectly. In fact, there is simply no medicine that can kill the viruses attacking humans; the only weapon we can wield against them is our immune system. This is evident from the fact that the treatment against viral fever is just to take supplements for your system while your immune system fights its battle. Almost (except for a few exceptional cases) every human is born with a strong immune system but throughout life, we tend to ignore the body's triggers and eventually our system gives upon us. This has become a norm in recent days resulting in different forms of sickness and even deaths. People die just because of a fever, which is a very sad thing to acknowledge.

In the past decade alone, we have seen a series of outbreaks including Avian Influenza, H1N1, Yellow fever, Dengue, Ebola and the list keeps going on. The most recent one that is shaking the whole world is the COVID-19 (also known as Corona Virus). It has become a norm to have an outbreak nowadays and, unfortunately, the most proven effective way to counter these kinds of outbreaks to vaccinate oneself. The vaccination gives a heads up to our immune system to prepare itself for an enemy intrusion. The most common form of vaccination subdues the original virus that causes the illness and inserts it into our own body under controlled conditions to give a feel of real danger to our immune system. Based on the subdued threat, our immune system comes up with the actual solution to manage a real intrusion. See how powerful and resourceful our immune system is! So all that one has to do is maintain a good relationship with our own body and keep our immune system in a top form always. It's like having a war general who would always obey you without doubts. As long as our body listens to our command, you can simply heal yourself and recover from any form of sickness.

Talking of outbreaks, I urge you to ask one simple question to yourself. When a single-celled organism like a virus can threaten the existence of multi-celled organisms like us, why should you be scared? It's like a single individual goes against an army of soldiers coordinated by a super-smart commander and suddenly the whole army of soldiers loses hope falling prey to this single individual. As improbable as it sounds but this is the reality when we face an infection from a foreign body. The single most prominent threat is always the fear of the enemy. This fear is worse than the enemy itself. In recent days, with the advancements in communication and media, this fear is multiplied beyond propositions. Slowly, every human succumbs to this darkness of fear and your body loses the capabilities to fight back a simple intrusion. This infection slowly spreads and brings down the whole system. I would leave the question hanging to hear as it will be best if the answer to this question is searched at one's efforts.

There are a few principles we should follow to make sure our body listens to us.

Sleep

Sleep is very important to regulate most of our body functions and the immune system is very much dependent on this fact. Even in a real war, the general need good sleep to plan and execute his next move against enemies; how is our immune system any different? Sleep is the time when you give your body enough time to assess the situation and overhaul itself. During sleep, every organ works at full force. When a person gets enough sleep, his body prepares with 100% efficiency for the next day.

> **"Your sleep quality is directly proportional to your physical and mental efficiency."**

How much amount of sleep a person requires solely depends on the individual itself. All that one has to do is listen to the body's triggers. Sometimes, we tend to oversleep and sometimes we are deprived of sleep. The primary factor that determines your quality of sleep is your habits.

> **"Harnessing deep sleep is a boon in childhood and later it becomes a skill to be mastered."**

The number of hours of sleep per person varies from six to nine hours. It depends on age, gender, environment and mindset. Nevertheless, the average human needs at least six hours of sleep a day to revitalize him. The other benefit of sleep is that it can relieve you from any form of stress, both physical and mental. And because of this enhanced mode of bodily functions, your immune system works best when you follow a regular sleep schedule. One of the most effective ways to improve sleep is to maintain sleep timings. If you suffer from sleep deprivation, it's time you take it seriously and find a solution, so that you achieve both peace and longevity because sleep is of utmost importance for maintaining health.

Rest

Most people don't differentiate between sleep and rest. Rest is giving you a break for a short duration of time, whereas sleep is the extended duration of a resting phase, which runs into hours. Like sleep, it is important to get a good amount of rest in a day. Rest is very important as well because the body does not need to wait till night to sleep to rejuvenate itself. When you give your body a temporary resting phase, it rejuvenates itself without waiting for a sleep process. It is like giving a short break between two intensive badminton games rather than closing the whole session. If you keep playing continuously, your system will shut down eventually. Let's take the computer as an analogy to understand the difference between shutdown and restart of a computer. A restart can resolve most of the application errors without the need for a full shutdown. It is quite fast and you get to operate the system without loss of time. An actual shutdown is also needed but only when the immediate needs have been rectified. Similarly, we need to give momentary rest to our system in the form of naps, meditation, good breathing exercises, leisure walks or any other form of related sorts.

Let's talk about a normal process of hospitalization or any form of rest advised by a medical practitioner. By right, if the medications are to cure your illness, you should return to your normal activities the moment you take the medicines but on the contrary, most of the patients are advised to rest for a period based on the seriousness of their condition. If you pursue further on this thought, you will arrive at an interesting answer. Our body needs rest to repair itself; however, not all forms of rest mean sleep. Even lying on a bed without spending your efforts on any other action is rest. This is much needed by our body to bring you back to normal form. If you observe closely, any form of sickness will try to put you down first and it's not the sickness itself but it is your own body telling you that it needs to concentrate its efforts on countering the sickness rather than any other activity. So all that you should do is, let your body do the work while you rest. When your body can repair itself during a resting period in the event of an injury or sickness, imagine what the body can do when you give rest at perfect intervals. Your overall health will significantly improve; this process of improving a particular condition is possible only when there is enough time and resources at the disposal of our own body. If you stick to a hectic schedule while you are in good health condition and only take rest while you are sick, then your body will get time only to fix the problem and not improve the condition. The best way to improve your overall health is to invest your time in yourself by allocating time for rest, sleep and relaxing activities daily.

We will see a few well-known processes that have been proven to provide significant health benefits.

Nap

A nap in the middle of a hectic workday will do wonders for your health. It gives your system a much sought after relief from the stress build-up. A nap improves your mental alertness and is known to improve the mood of a person. A person who takes a nap regularly is less prone to make mistakes mainly because of the mental alertness that follows after the nap period. Nap gives a sense of elation because you tend to forget all your immediate stress-causing emotions. This process rejuvenates your whole body and it tends to keep you sharp for the rest of the day. But a nap is effective only if it's for a short duration (less than 30 minutes). Usually, nap after lunch is the right time because of the following reasons.

- Lunchtime is at the middle of the day where you have already spent half of all your energy synergized during the night's sleep and it is the right time for short reloads of your energy levels.

- After a good meal, your body tends to focus your energy on digesting the meal and you will be functioning with less efficiency. Instead of trying to divert all your energy on your current task, it would be wise to give your body a temporary break so that it can perform digestion faster and fill you up with energy for the rest of the day.

- Nap towards the end of the day would disturb your night sleep cycle, which is not advisable.

Based on a study by NASA, a nap is proven to improve the efficiency of a person by 34%. Realizing this certain companies in Japan have introduced nap rooms within their office premises wherein their employees can take a nap for a short time and return to work fully recharged. No wonder the average Japanese lifespan is much better than the rest of the world.

If you still doubt the benefits of a nap, please try it once and you will instantly understand the benefits.

I am sure in recent days almost all big companies have recreational areas for their employees and it will be prudent to make the best use of it, a nap would be a good start.

Meditation

There are many different forms of meditation. I have had the privilege to learn four different forms of meditation, even though every form has its way of doing things, the underlying principle remains the same. You tend to give your mind a form of break from its constant state of thoughts. Our mind is the most powerful tool.

"Fear the one who sharpens his mind every day than the one with the sharpest sword."

The benefits of meditation are enormous and it has been repeatedly communicated through numerous successful people. The one thing I would like to emphasize is more than the psychological benefits the physical benefits of meditation are tremendous. Meditation is the time when your conscious mind scans the body for any form of weakness and in most cases, helps the body heal itself. Not only that we will be looking at the power of mindset in the coming chapters and meditation will help you focus your mindset on the right things.

In meditation, the emphasis is made on concentrating your conscious on your pain or any form of disturbance in specific and when you follow it correctly the pain and the disturbance disappears. I have personally had this experience. How can this be possible? I did a lot of research and finally concluded that the healing was done by our body and all that meditation was doing is just pointing out the exact pain area to our body just like you do with your doctor when he performs his diagnosis. There are a few differences between a doctor's treatment and our body's own healing capacity.

Doctor's Treatment Method	Body Healing Method
Relies on your account of what happened and so he proceeds with further tests to confirm his diagnosis.	Reconfirms your account of your conscious story with your subconscious, which is the most accurate one.
Treatment will take some time because the medicine has to be absorbed into our body for processing before it can perform its action.	It is internal and the effects are immediate, one another reason why the pain disappears even before you complete your meditation.
Charges you the fees based on the condition.	Absolutely free!

All I suggest is you should start looking at this angle of your body healing once in a while.

Toxins

Toxins are a stumbling block to any of our body functions. They are like obstacles on the road leading to health and longevity. A toxin here means the substances that accumulate within a human body and over time disrupt the functioning of various organs. Toxins don't necessarily have to come from the intake of poisonous substances or a bite from a poisonous animal. There are two methods by which toxins accumulate in our bodies.

- **The food we consume:** In recent days, most of the food we consume has added artificial substances, which tend to accumulate in our body. The reason is our body has been made to process natural elements and when an unnatural compound enters our digestive system it doesn't know what to do, so it simply stores it in our body without processing it. Imagine what will happen when you pump kerosene into a petrol vehicle. Something similar happens to our bodies.

- **Our eating habits:** Our bad eating habits have evolved over the decades resulting in an unhealthy environment for our body. We tend to eat fast to keep up with the fast-moving world but in essence, we are defeating our purpose of survival. That's the reason why I have explained the basic principles of eating habits in the previous chapter on food. By adopting those habits, one might reduce the intake of toxins but it is impossible to eliminate toxins from our food in this so-called advanced era.

Now, we need to understand the fact that toxins are going to be accumulated over a while; also, the more toxins in your body, the more trouble you are inviting to yourself. (Cancer is a classic example of sickness resulting due to the accumulation of toxins). So what can we do about the toxin problem? We need to adopt techniques to flush out the toxins from our bodies at regular intervals to maintain good health. Let's look at certain methods for toxin removals. These methods might be common across the world but the exact procedure that is followed varies depending on cultural differences and geographical factors.

Sweat it Out

Sweating is our natural way of releasing toxins from our bloodstream. In olden days, we never had the luxury of air conditioning and our sweating process was normal. And people then were accustomed to outdoor activities rather than indoors, since gadgets had not taken over their lives yet. No wonder our forefathers had a healthier life in spite of very little technological advancement. The more time we spend outdoors, the more we sweat and thereby expel the toxins regularly. It is perfectly normal for humans to evolve and invent new things but at the same time, we shouldn't forget the need for a few ways that can keep us healthy. You should make it a point to be involved in some form of outdoor activities, which can help you sweat out toxins from your body.

Purge Yourself

Purging is an activity of cleaning one's digestive tract. Based on Siddha form of medicine, it is suggested to purge the whole digestive system once in six months or at least once a year. Purging removes all the solid wastes accumulated within the digestive track over the years. It greatly helps in revitalizing your gut by cleaning it up. It helps in digestion, effective absorption of nutrients from our daily food and also enhances the expelling of solid wastes from our body. If you want to convince yourself of the importance of this process, you can talk to a patient suffering from constipation or discuss the effects of constipation with your medical consultant. Then, I strongly recommend you talk to a dietician or medical practitioner to guide you on the correct steps. This is another essential step in maintaining good health.

Get a Massage

Yes. Getting a good massage is also a very good way to flush out toxins from your body. As silly as it might sound, a proper massage tends to correct the flow of energy inside your body or streamlines the blood flow. When the flow happens, it breaks all the toxins stuck within your body and brings it to our toxin eliminating system—the kidneys. Our kidneys, in turn, remove these toxins through different forms of excretion. Most of the massage sessions will end up with a form of warm water intake or simple tea. In general, liquid intake is needed after every massage. The reason behind it is that our body needs water intake to flush out the toxins. The massage techniques help this liquid intake to circulate throughout our body accumulating toxins from the deep corners of our body and finally bring it to our kidneys for flushing. The massage is usually followed by a hot water bath; the reason behind as long as your body is warm the flow continues and a cold water bath might affect this flow.

Whenever a rusted iron pipe needs to be cleaned of its rust, we use hard surface paper or a metal brush to break and clean the rust powder. Similarly, massages break the toxins accumulated in our body like rust and expel them out of our body. How often to go for a massage depends entirely on the type of massage you avail. You can simply ask your masseur and they will be happy to help you with that part. In some cultures, massage is still not recognized as a way of life but eventually, it will become an integral part of people's search for health solutions.

Takeaways

- Connect with Mother Nature

- Feel the sun

- Trust your partner for life

Mindset and Emotions

Any situation can be looked at differently solely based on the attitude or mindset of the person looking at it. Every situation has both positive and negative angles. A positive attitude is synonymous with broad thinking, strong and expandable character. Likewise, a negative attitude is synonymous with narrow thinking, weak and confused character. If you look closely, every successful person will fall under the positive mindset category. So one way to be successful is just to change the way you see the world, this is the baseline message in most of the self-help books.

Let me tell you one of my real-life experiences to clearly understand the difference between the two attitudes. In my early 20s, I started developing a medical condition; I used to have stomach upset at least once a month sometimes even more than twice. It usually starts with mild stomach pain and will continue for three-four hours of vomiting, diarrhoea and stomach spasms. It would mostly happen during the bedtime and extend until early mornings. I visited several doctors and tried different kinds of medications. They gave me only temporary relief. This affected my sleep routine, and eventually had psychological repercussions. I was getting frustrated every time this incident happened to me. I went for food control measures against my desire to try varieties of cuisines. Whatever I tried was futile, and I came back, draining my physical and mental energy. After trying so many methods, the final relief came from a wellness therapist; the only treatment he gave was he asked me to look at the problem from a different perspective. He just opened my eyes to the brighter side of the problem; he showed me that I was looking at it all from the wrong perspective.

He said, "You don't need treatment for this condition because you have an internal dietician who is telling you that every time you eat something, which your body can't digest, it is pushing those unwanted things outside your system, and it is reminding you not to do it again. If this internal dietician doesn't tell you this, your system will be a pile of unwanted toxins and you will end up with something worse, causing permanent and serious damage."

Initially, when I heard this, I felt angry. I had a suspicion about the effectiveness of the doctor, who instead of giving me medicines for physical discomfort was asking me to change my attitude. At that moment I couldn't see the real message because of my physical and mental discomfort but later on after a day or so when I was in a clear state of mind I researched and found out that it was a blessing in disguise. The most common medical condition that occurs because of toxin accumulation is cancer. Well after that instance I always feel better whenever I throw up or have diarrhoea because I know the toxins are being expelled from my body. This change in attitude changed everything for me. Eventually, over time I had improved my food habits to make sure I only consume foods that my body accepts. And whenever someone asks how I found out, which food is accepted by my body, I used to smile and say, "It's simple. I try out different food items and if it gets expelled, then I mark it as bad for my body because my internal dietician has said so."

I know it's quite tough to change one's perspective over things especially when it is already haunting that person physically or mentally or both but just give a try once to search for the brighter side of things. I am sure you will be able to find a better solution to the problem.

This positive attitude towards life is so contagious that once you are infected with this, you will see that it will spread into all the aspects of your life. It will become your nature to start looking at the brighter side of everything. A positive-minded person will look at any form of a problem as an experience and will do all that is in his power to make sure he/she never faces a situation like that in life again by bettering himself, whereas a negative person will blame everyone and everything that has brought him/her to that situation while doing nothing worthy about the actual problem, simultaneously going down in his values.

Maybe it might look like this is all got to something with mind and emotions. If you feel so then you are grossly mistaken, anything that happens inside your thoughts will have a direct impact on your health. In the olden days, this fact was well understood by the medical practitioners who would always put in good words and faith in their patients first. These words do wonders on the patients, more evident on children than on adults because as you grow up you are trained only to look at facts and as per science the sickness is cured only by chemicals. If you notice, a sick child's condition dramatically improves the moment he/she is in the hospital and almost 70% are cured when the doctor smiles at them, saying a few good words. This is called the magic of mindset—the doctor just manages to change the mindset of the patient and the sickness automatically takes a backseat.

In all the forms of natural medicine, this is the ground rule for treatment. The first thing the practitioner addresses is the patient's mindset and only when he is convinced the person has a positive mindset over the sickness does the doctor considers the actual medicines. Furthermore, as per science, our body is made up of chemical elements and the sickness occurs when there is an imbalance in one of the elements. The sickness is treated by providing the chemicals to substitute the imbalance. If this is true, then there is one another proved fact that negative mindsets like stress, anger, anxiety and a few others affect our actual physical health because they disturb our internal hormone balance. If a negative mindset can affect our physical health, then a positive mindset should be able to heal the body. This is the point to be understood beyond doubt.

Creation Vs. Destruction

The world is made in such a way that the creation process is slow whereas destruction is instant. This applies to anything and everything. For example, building a house takes few months to years, while breaking it takes only a day; it takes years for a seed to transform into a tree, whereas only a few minutes to chop it down; creating a habit takes days whereas breaking it takes only a moment and this rule can be applied across a lot of things. Likewise, if you apply this rule to medical conditions, a person should take a longer time to heal than the time taken for the sickness to put you down. Based on this, you should be able to find the right type of approach for recovering from any illness.

Remember, as long as you go by the law of nature, it rewards you beyond your imagination. It will only take an instant to start believing in a positive attitude and taking your steps towards longevity. The age-old saying "Whatever happens happens for good" means the same but most of us don't see the bright side until later on when we connect the dots.

Having said that, adopting a positive attitude will be one of the best things to go about; it all depends on how well you can train your mind to look at the positive side of things. Initially, it will be a humongous task because all this while we have been taught to forget about this side of life. Our current education system, mass communication systems, entertainment shows mostly showcase the negative side of life because it's a universal truth that negative things affect people's emotions quite stronger than the positive ones. It is evident from the fact that people enjoy shows that showcase the negative aspects of a human than the show, which showcases positive aspects. If you deeply notice, most of the addictive TV series termed as blockbusters are based on the amount of light it can throw on the negative aspects of humans, for example, look at shows which are based on deception, lust and genocide and so on. I am not saying you should stop watching these shows or condemn them for good but reduce your addiction towards these kinds of series. You can always look into a comedy show or motivational talk once in a while.

Love the "No" Sayers

Irrespective of where you are, what position you hold, how many skills you possess the moment you start something new—be it a new project or new learning—the first person you may meet, mostly, will be the 'no' sayer. This person will be able to point out the possible failures in your new venture almost instantly. And the discussion ends with a 'no' to your efforts. This negative thought can bring you down despite all your positive motivations. You can't avoid them and the only way to overcome this problem is to start accepting them and tackling it from a positive angle. Whenever a person under this category shares with his thoughts don't fight it, instead, try to look at the root of the issue, taking out all the negative bias. This will help you to prepare yourself for the worst-case possibilities. The most relevant example will be when you fall sick, most of the messages that you will get will be on the worst-case scenarios, whereas if you just dig deeper, they will form only a fraction of the actual cases. Say you are down with a fever, most of your friends will remind you of the cases involving viral fever, which turned fatal, jaundice that took a toll on the patient's health permanently, some cases of Swine flu, which caused much suffering, etc. You might have just had a normal fever and it would take only take your body a day or two to recover completely but imagine the mental turmoil you would undergo during those two days not knowing what could go wrong.

That is something you can avoid by keeping a positive attitude.

For that matter, even if it's very high fever there are quite a lot of people who have recovered from the brink of fatality, all you need is to believe in yourself and never give up on hope. All your body needs to recover is hope and positive surroundings, which I have already indicated in the previous chapters of this book. You would be familiar with the nitro booster modes in racing games, which you can use to give an extra push. Likewise, if you train yourself to handle these 'no' sayers, in a matter of time, they will become the nitro boost that pushes your forward. You start seeing them as a challenge and will set yourself on a track to prove them wrong. This is my personal experience and I started loving these 'no' sayers for the boost they give me every time I face a hurdle or start something new. I hope you also start loving them.

Purpose

Every living thing on earth has to have a purpose; without purpose, life doesn't hold any meaning. Discovering the purpose of life is the most important thing in a person's life. What is it going to do with longevity? Let's assume you are travelling in a car and your destination is your purpose. What happens if you are driving a car without knowing the destination? You will simply be following the road in whichever direction it turns and finally you won't reach anywhere. End of the day, the car's fuel, your energy and the whole journey would have been a complete waste. That's why you should know your purpose or at least adopt one. If you don't have a purpose eventually you will end up following someone else's path, in some cases it may turn out to be the best decision of your life provided you chose the right one to follow. If your choice was wrong then obviously you would have wasted your life on the wrong choice. So it's always better to have a purpose of your own to have a successful life. Having a successful life and longevity are very much related. If you look back at our history and even the present, successful people are ones who tend to live longer.

Even though good scientific reasons connect successful life with longevity, the simplest explanation can be through an example. When a person plays every day, whatever game he chooses, say, badminton, his or her game improves gradually and mastering the game will take years. If that same person trains with the purpose of participating and winning a tournament, the time taken to master the game is considerably reduced. Not only does he save time, but his capabilities also improve significantly as well. This is a very important principle that can be applied across any area of our life.

Now, in the above example, you can substitute badminton with fitness, professional work, personal relationships, longevity or any other life's attribute. You will start seeing considerable changes as long as you can attach a purpose to your actions. This is very evident among the most successful persons in the world.

One of the most notable differences between an extraordinary person and a normal person is his attitude towards life.

> **"Either you should have the guts to copy someone or at least should have the talent to create on your own."**

Emotions

Prepare for battle! Ready your weapons!

One of my childhood interests was martial arts. I have had the opportunity to learn three different fighting forms under great masters. Over this period, I was made to understand one concrete fact—a weapon is a liability or asset based on who wields it, which has absolutely no relevance to the weapon itself. This rule applies to our everyday lives. We are fighting our own battles every day and there are weapons, which you hold with or without your knowledge during these battles. The idea is to understand these weapons and make better use of them.

Take precautions! The weapons we are going to discuss now are the strongest known to mankind and the one who can master all of them will be indomitable. We will be looking at four weapons—happiness, fear, humiliation and love. Yes, every emotion we feel is a powerful weapon if you know how to control and wield it. Emotional control is a skill that needs to be learned and mastered by practice. Unlike the physical weapons, which you use in a real fight to attack your opponents, these emotional weapons are to be used on oneself to improve, succeed in a task, heal oneself, even survive a fatal condition, or achieve great health. In our everyday life, we face numerous challenges and you will feel different emotions, each one having an impact on your health. As long as they are your liability, you tend to lose everything because as I have already mentioned earlier—health is everything. The better you become in handling theses emotions, the more you will celebrate your daily challenges and in time, you will start celebrating longevity.

Emotional Weapons

Emotions are bound with mindset but the basic difference is that emotions are a state of mind at an instant, whereas mindset is how you control your reaction to emotional stimuli. Handling emotions forms an important part of maintaining a healthy mindset and body. Emotions are also classified as positive and negative emotions. Unlike mindset, I wouldn't say we should have only positive emotions because it is human nature to have both positive and negative emotional stimuli. We will only look at how to respond to these emotional stimuli. There are a few very strong emotions as discussed above that can push us to break our limits. Those are the emotions that you should invoke to push yourself towards longevity.

Happiness

There isn't a soul in this world that wouldn't want to be happy. Happiness can get you out of any form of trouble. Happiness decides the quality of one's life. If there is one thing that everyone should get daily, then I would say it should be a dose of happiness. There is no equal medicine for this momentary feeling and there is no illness it can't cure. What makes a person happy? This question can be answered best internally only by each individual to oneself. So the first thing that you can do is to write down a list of things that makes you happy and find out ways that can be repeated every day. It could be a person, relationship, TV shows, books or activity. Based on whichever suits you, do plan in such a way that you get a good dose of happiness at least once a day. With this miraculous potion, you can push your lifespan over bounds.

This will be evident whenever you have a chance to chat with those above 70 years of age or kids below six years, the most remarkable quality that you will identify will be their sense of humour. There is a saying from my grandparent's time,

"Spend time with children (young and elderly) every day to know happiness!"

There aren't words to explain the feeling one will have when you go through that experience. My suggestion is you should try it at least once in life. Here's a light-hearted joke:

Million Dollar Reply

Friend 1: On the way to the workout venue, hurrying through the traffic posted a message to her workout mates "I am running late, reaching the venue in 10 minutes. Which floor is the practice?"

Friend 2: Cement floor.

Friend 1: ?????

I used to hear my grandparents saying, **"A heart full of laughter will cure any pain."**

This is true. This is because the happy hormones secreted in our body when we laugh have a lot of healing effects on the body. This has been recently identified. Thus laughter therapy is gaining momentum in hospitals, wherein they deliberately take efforts in making the patient happy and also make them laugh. There is even a form of forcefully induced laughter therapy wherein a person is forced to imitate laughing, this therapy is not as effective as the naturally occurring laughter but it does help. The easier way to adapt to this medicinal therapy is to take a note of everyday happy moments in a diary or notebook or even in your mobile and try to go through them whenever you feel low. You will see that your mood and health significantly turns better. Based on human psychology, our mind remembers occasions by relating it to recent memory and so the more you remind yourself of the happy moments, the better you will feel. This is one of the key values to possess for longevity.

Follow the guidelines that are listed below whenever you feel pain, either physical or mental.

1. Close your eyes and sit in a calm place.

2. Remember the last time you laughed out loud and try to recollect the vivid experiences that made you do that.

3. Relish the experience one more time in your mind.

4. Now open your eyes and see if you still feel the pain.

My experience tells me your pain will be either reduced to the extent that it doesn't disturb you anymore or it would have completely disappeared.

Fear

Fear is another emotional stimuli that can affect all your senses at the same moment. This emotion is mostly mishandled by a lot of people.

> **"Fear of failure can create great success."**

Once my school topper was asked to address the students by our principal in our assembly. She was expected to re-emphasize our principal's motto "Study every day." Surprisingly her speech made us think in a different dimension. Her secret of success was her fear of exams; in spite of her fears, she studied only on the day before the exams. Every student will have a fear of exams but she had increased her quantum of fear by postponing the studying part till the day before the exam. It meant she start studying a subject book only on the day or two before the actual exam. By following this particular step, her focus during the exam study was concrete and she just had to study a particular topic once or max twice. That was enough for her mind to remember the subject. Initially, she had to follow it because of circumstances but later on she developed it as a habit. This particular habit improved her concentration skills tremendously. She went on to prove her concentration skills through different competitions. Unwillingly or willingly, she has converted her fear stimuli in her favour.

This is similar to a scenario where a normal person having difficulty walking will transform himself into a sprinter when pursued by a street dog. Fear becomes a trouble only when it is not addressed over a period of time. In the above example if the person outruns the dog then he will appreciate his own physical abilities. When he doesn't manage to outrun, the dog will become his obsession for the rest of his life or till the point when he faces his own fear. The key point in handling this emotion is to accept the fear and doing something about it.

Fear not handled properly will lead to dejection and negative emotions. Any form of fear can be overcome if proper methods are followed. Without fear of death, there won't be any reason for humans to pursue health and longevity at such proportions. So it is perfectly normal to be scared; just accept it and use this emotion to move forward.

Humiliation

"There is no real achievement without suffering."

Humiliation is a momentary experience that will have long-lasting effects. Usually forgetting this momentary experience is the toughest challenge one can face. The following reaction will be one of anger, revenge, depression or all of them. In general, humiliation is one of the negative emotions because it is felt when someone's weaker side is exploited by another person, eventually hurting the person at a psychological level. Humiliation usually leaves a scar for life in most scenarios. Most of us will be able to recollect the vivid experiences of humiliation even after a considerable number of years have passed. The reason is that it is a very strong emotion that can stimulate all your senses at the same time. Usually, such an experience gets registered in our subconscious memory without much effort. Once an experience is registered in your subconscious memory, it takes a lot of effort to erase it. Our conscious memory is like the words written on a whiteboard with a marker, whereas subconscious memory is like the words written on a whiteboard marker with a permanent marker. The later can't be erased off so easily and it requires special efforts like meditation, counselling, hypnotism or other ways of similar sorts.

Even though humiliation is a negative feeling if we wield this emotion in a positive way, the results will be dramatic. The good side of this emotion is that it gets registered at our subconscious level without much effort from our side. The usual purpose that one relates to humiliation is to exact revenge on the person or thing that has caused this feeling. A normal person will resort to violence or some sort of destructive means to avenge this feeling but if you think through there won't be much relief even after that. So what do we do? How do we deal with this humiliation? There are two ways that I can share at this point—one, you can choose to forget the incident by taking special efforts, which are mostly advised by the learned and experienced people. Two, I encourage you to try to go back into avenging mode, to that burning feeling, but in a positive way.

> **"The best way to exact revenge is by proving that you can be better."**

Let's look at a small story to understand this more clearly. There was this schoolboy who was 12 years of age. He was the class's favourite for all forms of bullying because he was the shortest in class and also he didn't have any attractive features as well. This went day after day until he could no longer bear. Imagine the humiliation that he would have felt when every day in school he was bullied and called all sorts of names reminding him of his shortcomings. Since he was still a school goer, he didn't have many choices to retaliate offensively. Noticing that this kid was becoming more and more disturbed at home, his dad sat with him and after a long chat, he realized the issue. And a usual dad's reaction would be to report this incident to the respective school authorities and take it head-on with the other kid's parents. But his dad took a different approach; he took his son and went over to a karate school near his house and made him join the class. Additionally, instead of consoling his son he gave him a stern look and said,

"It's your problem and you have to deal with it; neither me nor your mom for that matter not even God would help you on this. If you want to survive in this world better yourself and stand your ground against your oppressors."

That was a turning point in that kid's life and from that day, he started bettering himself every day. In a few months, he was the topmost student in his karate class and he went on to win his first championship in his age category. The day the news was out in the school, the atmosphere around him changed and all his oppressors became his supporters, may be out of fear or respect but his life changed over completely. Now even after years later this kid now a grown man is still serious about his karate practices and is one of the state's top karate champions. He is my close friend as well and sadly I was one of his oppressors. His fitness levels are way above his peers and no one even dares to bully him ever to this day.

Even today, whenever someone questions about his motivation behind his success, he would point to his humiliating experiences and how they make him go the extra mile every time he practices. One hell of a friend to have!!

The key point in this anecdote of my friend's success is that humiliation can be a strong motivation to better yourself in any aspect of life if you know how to wield it in the right way. So in your pursuit of longevity, I would suggest you imagine your sickness or your physical shortcomings as a humiliation and start motivating yourself to be better than that. Whenever you are sick just look yourself in the mirror, imagine the sickness causing bacteria or virus is in front of you and say out loud, "This is a humiliation to me because you have exploited my weakness but this will be the last time you get to do it. Next time, you dare not come near me for I will be too strong for you."

It will give you a motivational push to heal yourself and also pursue healthier habits. I am sure when you do it, you will end up with a healthier life and you won't need special efforts to motivate yourself over healthy habits. And one of the positive effects of this will be a longer lifespan.

Feel the Love

Love is one of the most strongly felt emotions among all the living things. It is not limited to just humans alone; every animal feels an emotion of love to another. This emotion is one another among the strongest, which can make you do things which you haven't imagined. If humiliation contributes to achievements, then love can contribute to the rest of it. Love is an equally strong emotion that can move the world. Imagine a mother trying to save her child from a predator, however indomitable the predator is the mother will still do all in her power to save her child whatever may be the consequences; this is an expression of true love. Few other forms of unadulterated love are also there, which can't be generalized into a single criterion.

When a person feels love towards another, he/she breaks boundaries to quantify this emotion and expect reciprocation. In this process, he/she would have achieved a lot more than what he/she would do under normal circumstances. The only sad part is that most of these successes are overlooked, as the primary motive still revolves around the person towards whom this emotion is targeted. This emotion is so powerful that a few who never receive the reciprocation resort to extreme measures, including ending one's own life. This is the part where one should become aware of the power behind this emotion: if a person can do so much for another person why can't the same emotion be contributed to bettering oneself in the form of self-love?

Whenever you have to talk to successful people, the one thing that will be very obvious is the self-love they feel towards themselves. They love themselves more than anyone in the world, which is why they better themselves every time trying to achieve greater limits feeling more happiness than before. This form of emotion can give you the power to cure yourself of any form of sickness and suffering; all you have to do is understand the love you deserve. Most of the successful billionaires also benefit themselves from this singular emotion, which will be evident when you read their biographies or listen to their stories.

A word of caution though is that some take it a little far towards selfishness, which has a recoil effect. Usually, selfishness backfires on oneself with negative effects. Hence, it is important to understand the difference between the two and strive towards betterment. There is a hairline difference between self-love and being selfish. Being selfish is an extreme form of self-love, wherein one wants to achieve results at the cost of another person.

Self-Love: Clear mindset, happiness, better relationships

Selfishness: Troubled mindset, sadness, unstable relationships.

Attitude Vs. Emotions

There is an invisible bond between the attitude of a person and the emotions he feels. It takes time to understand this bond and it is a magical bond that can grant you wishes far beyond your imagination. The better you understand this, the higher your chances of achieving health and longevity. This is one of the reasons why almost all the life coaching sessions will target adjusting your attitude for better as they know the moment you change your attitude, everything changes in life. For example, a person with a significant positive attitude always feels positive emotions like happiness and love while the person with a negative attitude feels more of negative emotions like anger and humiliation. This positive feeling is not limited to your health alone; one of the most important points that every wealth guru will tell you is to change your attitude towards money. Similarly, it is very important to train your mind to adopt a positive attitude, thereby enriching your life with positive emotions. The more positivity you have in life, the more you want to live on and you will start enjoying life with all its colours.

Takeaways

- Have a positive mindset

- Define a purpose for yourself

- Wield your emotions appropriately

Relationships

Without relationships, there will be no meaning to human evolution. We have evolved so much because of our ability to form relationships with other humans, animals and even nature. Relationships could be as simple as an acquaintance or a very special one like a soul mate. The basic requirement for a relationship is to appreciate the value of other entities. Relationships are quite important for one to improve. If there were no relationship there wouldn't be any life now because as per the popular myth the first human relationship started with Adam and Eve; without them, there wouldn't be any human life on earth. A relationship is a complex psychological process and usually, it involves a lot of emotions both happy and sad.

But we must look into relationships, for it is the relationship that decides the quality of life. We wouldn't be looking at all the possible relationships that exist, as I don't have the expertise in relationship management. Here are some forms of relationships that can help you on your path towards longevity.

You need a family to have a life.

You need friends to enjoy your life.

You need enemies to achieve in life.

"Family supports you, friends help you and enemies motivate you!"

For a few lucky ones, family and friends are almost the same. Their family will form a major part of their friends or their friends will become their family. The common differentiating factor is the amount of trust that revolves around a particular relationship. The moment you consider a person a friend, it means he/she has gained a part of your trust. If this trust evolves and you put all your trust over a particular relationship, then this relationship is termed as family. Usually, the family relationship refers to the blood relationships but I would prefer to define family relationships as the one where you share complete trust. Friendship is slightly lower but still, they form a crucial part of our lives. The general perception is that having enemies is a bad thing but I prefer you to look into this relationship from a different angle. You will be able to comprehend this point of view when you have read this whole chapter.

Friendship is one of the utmost important relationships we need in our life. There can be people without family but we rarely come across people who don't have a friend. Friends are categorized based on how well you know that person and how much trust one has on another. Gaining the trust of a person is the toughest task in any relationship. For the family, it is a given thing.

Additionally, relationships are like the rope that you use to secure yourself while trying an adventurous activity (imagine bungee jump, deep cave dive, mountain climbing, etc.). This rope helps to pull you back from any kind of adversity. Without this rope, you simply cannot exist. Similarly, when faced with adversity, you need strong relationships to pull you back into life. Some relationships are so strong that they can pull you out of a fatal condition; you need to feel a strong relationship to understand this one.

"True relationships are the ropes that can pull you out of any adversity."

So please make sure you have at least one or two strong ropes to secure your life.

Along with that, you need to understand different categories of relationships to better your chances of survival. Below is a certain way of classifying relationships.

Relationship Categories

All the relationships can be categorized under one of the blocks mentioned below. Like any pyramid structure, the below pyramid highlights the ideal proportion of the relationship categories for a happy and healthy life.

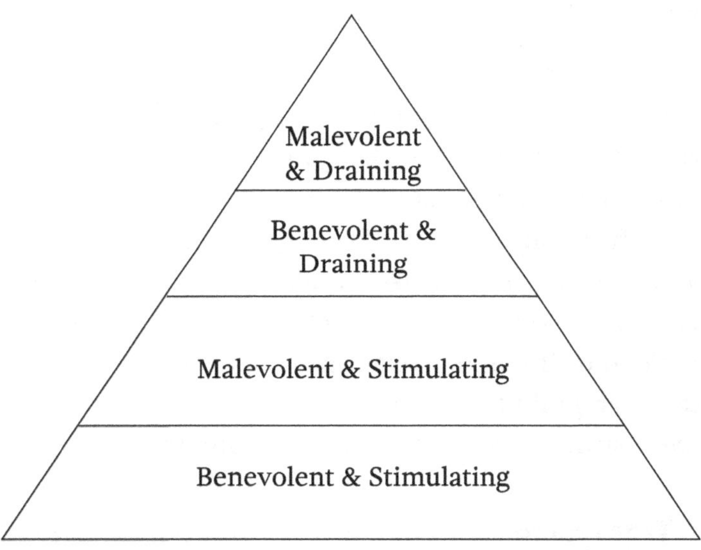

Malevolent and Draining

This type of relationship is very easy to find among almost all walks of life. The best example of this kind of relationship is when someone is betrayed by another. These kinds of relationships don't do any good and mostly speaking to this kind of person will leave you feeling dull, tired and you will be loaded with negative emotions like anger, frustration at the end of the conversation. But you don't need to feel negative emotions towards that person. Common instincts when you are with this person will be to instigate your negative emotions on another person or thing, thereby indirectly ruining your emotional peace. Even if you do feel negative emotions, we have already seen how to use it for your own good in the previous chapter.

Benevolent and Draining

This is also a common form of relationship, which is not harmful but takes your time and effort. The weak-willed people or those who always need support most of the time fall under this category. Usually, these are the people with whom if you spend a considerable amount of time, you will feel tired and drained. It will happen casually; later on, you will feel like you have lost the energy to do the tasks that you had already planned. This is because the persons under this category are completely negative in life. Meaning, they tend to see the negative aspect of things most of the time and rarely see the brighter side. They tend to feel that life is unfair and they are the less privileged than others and don't count their blessings. Because of this, they need you to show them the positive side of things or at least console them during their hard times. These might be your friends with whom you move around every day. Once in a while, spending your efforts in helping this kind of person is good but if it is the case on a day-to-day basis, I suggest you reconsider your priorities. In the long run, you would have spent considerable time helping others instead of even yourself. It is a balance that you should bring in by believing a simple fact.

> **"You can help people only if they accept it."**

Usually, this category of people has a weak mindset. They don't involve themselves in many activities rather set an invisible boundary around them and try to stay within it. Nothing wrong having this kind of people around but they don't motivate you as they lack motivation. They are ready to help but not sure of how to do it. These are the kind of people who like to stay around with persons with strong will and determination in doing things. They tend to follow you as long as you value their relationships. They are like the boogies following the train engine and you will need to put in additional efforts to take them along in your success journey.

Malevolent and Stimulating

Your competitors will form a major part of this category and to some extent, even your enemies. Let's look at the competition side first; your performance will be valued based on your competition. Imagine Usain Bolt running a 100m dash alone in a race event, how much will you enjoy the race or for that reason how much do you think Mr. Bolt will enjoy participating in the event. You will need competition to motivate yourself towards higher limits. As I have already mentioned in the previous chapters, there is no fun in performing an activity all by yourself. You will have personal satisfaction only when you win a race or game with an equal competitor. Otherwise, it will just be a time-pass activity.

> **"Real fun lies in winning a game with an equal or better competitor."**

Looking at the enemies under this relationship category, like I already mentioned in the previous chapter regarding emotions, revenge is one of the strongest emotions that can push you long past your limits. A simple insult can leave a long-lasting memory and immense negative energy; if you learn to focus this energy on the positive side, then I am sure none can stop you from success.

For instance, if you are bullied based on your physical shortcomings, then make it a point to prove them wrong by achieving better health and strength. By doing so, you prove two things—one, you are triumphing over your oppressors and two, you are becoming healthier, thereby improving your quality of life. And once you start following good healthy habits, it is very unlikely that you will fall back to your old unhealthy habits.

Considering longevity as a race; you will need the right portion of your relationships to fall under this category.

Benevolent and Stimulating

This category of relationship is like the magical happy potion that you can consume almost anytime and every time. Your true friends and family, who would go to any extent to make sure you get the best that you deserve, fall under this category. Ironically, this kind of relationship is a little elusive and quite tough to find easily. Even though people think that most of their friends and family circle fall under this category, you will know for certain only when you are met with a crisis.

Anyone can be your friend when you are flourishing with wealth, health and happiness, the true point of this relationship can be learned only when you are seriously into trouble and at your wits' end. These kinds of people can steer you out of any kind of situation and will be a beacon of hope throughout your hard times. They support and motivate you in spite of your shortcomings. They do it because they value your relationship much more than their priorities. If you have at least one person falling under this category, then I will call you the luckiest.

You need to have caution, as the 'malevolent and draining' relationship people will mostly imitate this 'benevolent and stimulating' category of people because it is the easiest way to win one's trust. If you are looking to live long, I would strongly suggest you look forward to people who fall under this category. Just being with this kind of person will give you hope over any form of mental or physical illness. One of the well-established facts in the world is

> **"Hope is the best cure."**

Having seen the relationship classifications, you need to understand the essential point at this juncture. No relationship is perfect and the relationship evolves on its own. At any point in time, you can't have only one of the above-mentioned category people in life because life is quite complicated. You will have to accept the point that your relationships will always be a mixture of the above four categories and it's up to you to prioritize your relationships based on which best suits your lifestyle.

In this book, our goal is to achieve health and longevity. Having a smaller portion of the third category and higher portion of the fourth category people in your close circle of family and friends will play a vital role.

Do You Have a Pet?

Over time humans have proved that any living form of animal can be tamed to be pets. Generally, dogs, birds and cats form the major portion of the household animal. And scientific studies have proven beyond doubt that having a pet in the house has a positive impact on the family environment. Generally, females of a species are thought to be most perceptive of human emotions and so they can make you feel comfortable providing you find the right one. In certain cases though finding the right one is a tough task, for those falling in this category, I would suggest to buy or adopt a pet.

Pets are also very perceptive of human emotions and since their only priority in life is being with their loved ones, they make sure you feel good always. I have had the privilege to have dogs as pets from my childhood and it has had a significant impact on my emotions and my life as a whole. Since I am more into dogs, I will explain it from the view of a person who owns a pet dog but after further research, I found out that having a dog, cat or any other pet animal has the same effects.

Pets' first and last priority will always be their master. They eat, breathe and live only to be loved by their master and reciprocate the same love on their masters. You can't guarantee a 100% dedicated relationship from any other human because it's natural for everyone to have their priorities. Even your closest families, including your partner, will have priorities that they have to attend. But pets are always on your side. Pets make an ideal companion for someone who has just lost everything.

Research has proved that having a pet in the old age increases your lifespan, reduces the possibility of heart disease. All pet owners know and enjoy how when they open the door to go inside their house, the first soul waiting to greet them will always be their pet. Personally, when I enter my house, I always engage with my pup and he wouldn't rest until I have done so. However stressful my day would have been, 10 minutes with my pup releases all my stress, making me more open and positive. Pets are one of the strongest stress busters that one can get. For certain people they give them purpose, when you turn old, life becomes slower and you will have hardly anything to do, which will push you towards boredom. The ideal remedy to this situation will be to own a pet.

"Ideal mind is a devil's workplace and pets are the guardian angels who keep that devil away."

However, having a pet and having an animal in the house are two different things. Confused? What I mean is, if you treat your pet dog as a mere watchdog, assigning him only duties of fetching and safeguarding and not treating him as a household member, then you may not reap the full positive impact. In fact, it may even create a negative impact.

"Pet is a living creature, which is a part of your family."

For example, you buy a dog and assign it to its primary task of guarding the house and its master. You keep him tethered during the day and release him only during the night. You make sure he stays outdoors within his defined boundary most of the time. You walk him two times a day, feed him and take care of him. Does it mean you have a pet? It's a big NO. All that you will feel is an additional responsibility and a sense of untidiness, which are the shortcomings of any pet animal. You are just having an animal guarding the house; it is similar to having a guard outside your house. The latter option is still a better one.

In such a scenario, there is no emotion involved between you and your dog. You will become tired and even more frustrated with every passing day. All the above positive effects of having a pet are only felt when you make that animal a part of your family. As in the above example, if you let the dog move around without restrictions and you treat him like a family, then you won't feel any of the responsibilities like it's a burden, because it's like having a kid in your house. This is how you own a pet.

Not only the elderly need a pet the younger generations tend to learn a lot from having a pet in the house. A child's social behaviour improves if you have the right kind of pet in the house. The kids who grow up with pets understand emotions much better than the ones who don't. They are compassionate and responsible towards other kids, as they tend to learn by example. The pets shower the kids with love and in some cases more than their parents due to their tight work schedule. These kids tend to reciprocate the same love towards their friends and family. As I mentioned earlier, if your emotions are positive, your health will stay at its prime always.

So if you are thinking of buying a gift to your elderly parents or your kids do consider buying a pet that can suit your environment. They will surely guarantee you a good positive atmosphere.

Make Friends

Research on social relationships between people has revealed that a strong social relationship increases your chances of survival by 50%. I will completely agree with this because I strongly feel the most integral part of a healthy lifestyle is to make friends and stick to them. There could be many reasons why you want an acquaintance but converting an acquaintance into a friendship means sharing your trust with the other person. Let's say if you are to fall from a cliff into an abyss (a metaphor for bad health, economic downturns, personal losses, bad relationships, etc.), friends are the ropes around you who won't let that happen no matter what. The more ropes you have, the safer you are. If you feel this statement is overrated, walk over to the park for a week and observe the crowd. The regulars are always the ones with friends, whereas those who are on their own tend to disappear as time passes by. This is because they lack the motivation coming from a friend.

Most people realize the importance of friendship only towards the end because that is when they understand what matters in life. This is evident from the fact that most of the elderly people tend to make more friends than the younger ones.

There are two stages when you make friends who stick with you for life. Firstly, when you are a kid, your friends accept you for what you are rather than who you are; secondly, when you are retired, as they make friends who support each other rather than gain from each other.

It doesn't mean you can't make friends in the middle stages of your life; it's slightly biased by a lot of other factors like social status, economic conditions, which affects your decision of identifying the right person. If you are not convinced, ask how many of your friends are happy with their partners. Most of us select partners in an emotional rush and later realize the mistake, which often ends in the splitting of the relationship. Nevertheless, understanding your relationships and forming the right type of relationships always helps in mental health, which indirectly means a better happy life.

Takeaways

- Understand relationship categories

- Have a pet

- Make friends

Habits

"It is always hard to make or break a habit."

There is an invisible link between relationships and habits. This link defines the quality of your habits, habits, in turn, define your lifestyle, and lifestyle, in turn, defines your health, which in turn decides your lifespan. So this link is very important. Let's say you make a friend with interests in sports; there is a high probability your interest will slightly move towards sports as well. This is the power of social relationships. When you make friends from different walks of life, you tend to learn a lot through mutual sharing and also your quality of life improves tremendously. With every new relationship, your habits tend to change. You must choose the right kind of relationships though. The secret of success embarks on two important aspects: habits and relationships. We will look at a few habits, which have personally helped me and which I believe will help you as well.

Reading

This habit is one of the most effective and simple ones, which is overlooked by a lot of people.

> **"School books make you a responsible person; self-help books make you a successful person."**

This is well understood by all the successful people, which is why an average CEO reads around 50 books a year. The usual mistake that people make is, they believe that success in life means wealth and its derived factors. But one who doesn't enjoy proper health won't be able to enjoy his success. Do you think one can celebrate a success story from a hospital bed? Reading boosts up your knowledge, which is a well-established fact but reading also helps people maintain mental health. Reading every day is like exercising your brain, which is also a muscle. Every muscle needs exercise and if you don't exercise this muscle, you will start losing your senses as you age. Ailments resulting from ignorance of this fact include Alzheimer's, one of the deadliest diseases in recent times, where you simply forget everyone and everything around you and slowly, you forget yourself. After this point, there is not much meaning to your life. So remember to keep your brain in shape before worrying about your physical shape.

Reading has a few side effects as well; it can make you forget your troubles (of course, that depends on how much the book has engaged you), gives you purpose, kills boredom, brings friendship, etc. Personally, the quality of my life started taking an upward curve after I adopted this habit. And when it comes to reading it is entirely up to the individual to choose the type of book he reads. Some might like self-help, some novels, some news materials, and some specific science materials; irrespective of what you choose, reading is still a must-have habit for anyone.

Walking

Walking is one another undervalued habit and most of the time it is reserved for elders and sick persons. This is because of the ideas rooted in our belief systems. Initially, when a person is young, he/she would prefer a more active exercise like jogging, running or any other form of sports. The middle-aged ones simply don't find time for it and even if they do and if they are physically able, then they involve themselves in a more engaging activity. That leaves only the elders and sick persons who can't afford to do any of the active sports, who are advised to go for walking. By right, everyone should inculcate this habit in his or her lifestyle for a few reasons:

1. Walking gives a constant rhythm to your body; it is like taking your car on a smooth road for a drive. It gives a good feel along with improved blood flow to your whole body, which can

improve your chances against several ailments (including heart conditions, diabetes, stress, strokes, etc.).

2. Walking improves your social life because when you walk at regular times, you will meet people regularly and you tend to make good friends over a period of time.

3. Unlike any sports activity, there is no risk of injury and anyone can try it.

4. You get to be one with nature at least for some time, the importance of which has already been discussed in the previous chapters.

If you can't get yourself to walk every day, then get yourself a dog and then it will be your dog's responsibility to push you for a walk.

Run a Marathon

Running a marathon is the best thing that you can do to test your endurance (both physical and mental). The sense of achievement in running a marathon lies in the marathon itself rather than the medal you get when you complete it. Most of the people take a back seat when they hear the number of kilometres (precisely 42.195 km) one need to run a marathon. All they see is only the distance but if one can take a leap of faith and participate in the marathon, the experience will speak for itself.

I consider a marathon as a way to convince your soul that you have what it takes to face any challenge coming your way. This self-assurance is very much needed for every individual whenever they are tested by extreme conditions, especially physical sickness. The moment a person falls sick, the primary impact will be on one's mind irrespective of what the illness might be. I believe these disease-causing viruses and pathogens know this crucial fact that the key to their success in bringing down a human lies in the sole point of breaking the particular individual's will power to stop the invasion. There are a few ways to train oneself for such adversity but the easiest I know is just run a marathon. I am sure you will never regret your decision at any point in life.

When I took the leap of faith and registered for my first marathon, I was just 30 years old. I had this fear, which kept me awake during nights, especially when the days were running fast and I lacked the will to do any serious practice. I did practice a few times but never was I confident of completing the marathon. And how will I be? The longest distance I have run before that was just 15 km and this marathon was almost three times the same distance. I slept for hardly three hours on the previous night of the marathon. Fear kept me awake and I even considered withdrawing from the run.

But I went ahead and participated. For the first 10 km, I kept telling myself to reach the 15 km mark and then stop if I can't proceed. But when I touched the 12 km mark, a miracle happened. I was hardly jogging as my body was giving out signals in all forms of pain; at that instant, an elderly person overtook me and ran ahead. Then he turned back and gave a smile signalling his hand towards me. He was telling me to catch up with him. He did it for a few seconds and continued running, even though he never looked back I got this power surge inside me and for the rest of the 30 km, the only thing that kept me running was that person's smile and his simple gesture. It was like my body had received a supercharge and the pains weren't bothering me anymore. I was running, jogging, walking and the last few kilometres I had to limp my way towards the finish line, but I finally did it. I never had a chance to see that person again nor did we exchange words; it was that one moment when he came out of nowhere and became my lucky angel.

After completing that marathon, my tolerance towards pain in any form increased manyfold. I never had to worry about my illness and eventually, I saw very few physical illnesses thereafter. Even if there was a condition that brought me down, it lasted only for a short while and I bounced back to my peak health in a matter of a few hours. My recovery time from any form of illness was quite fast. I know quite a few scientific explanations that connect a marathon preparation and health but I don't feel the need to prove it here in this book. All I would like to emphasize is the magic that happened to me after my first marathon.

Now the above is my experience of mine comes with a **disclaimer,** running a full marathon comes with a lot of risks. So if you are planning to adopt this habit, then I suggest you start with a smaller distance, prepare yourself and then find your way to this ultimate experience.

Not just the marathon, even preparing for a marathon can be very rewarding. So what are you waiting for?

Similar to the marathon experience, the other way to enthral yourself is to test your skills in tough sports or to participate in a competitive sport or tournament of your choice. When you have forced yourself into a competitive environment, you indirectly challenge yourself and the result is still the same. The key point to note is getting yourself a challenge once in a while so that your physical and mental tolerance levels go up and stays at a good level that keeps you at your prime health conditions.

Takeaways

Cultivate Habits:

- Reading

- Walking

- Run a marathon/challenge yourself

Celebrate Life!

To sum things up, life is precious. So everyone should take health as a serious concern. Already, health awareness and wellness concepts are reaching large masses of people. Even the developing countries and underdeveloped countries are emphasizing on its importance in recent times. I hope this humble anecdote of mine would help a little more people become aware of the health and ways to achieve optimum health.

Also, a community's development depends on the people with age greater than 60 as they are the people who have survived the race of life and have time and knowledge to give back to the next generation. Only when this giving back takes place, the next generation will gain insight into important things in life and they can celebrate life. Currently, people still keep running in life even after 60 years (a few who never retire), few never see 60 due to health implications, and a few cross the 60 from a hospital bed. These people won't be able to pass on their life experiences to the next generation and this new generation again runs the same race accumulating the same knowledge through the hard way. The easiest way would be from the elders who share their experiences to the next generation.

At this point, I acknowledge the fact that everyone is unique and their problems are also unique. The methods that I have discussed here is to create awareness and get you thinking in the right direction. If the need arises, you can very well look for more specific solutions and maybe you will stumble upon something better. Every day new methods are being discovered for the betterment of humanity. When you do stumble upon some priceless insights, what will you do? I, sincerely, hope you make a conscious choice to share your knowledge with the world so that people can grow and become better.

Thank you for reading this book!